Tuberculosis: Challenges in Diagnosis and Management

Tuberculosis: Challenges in Diagnosis and Management

Edited by **Morris Beckler**

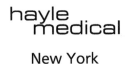

hayle
medical

New York

Published by Hayle Medical,
30 West, 37th Street, Suite 612,
New York, NY 10018, USA
www.haylemedical.com

Tuberculosis: Challenges in Diagnosis and Management
Edited by Morris Beckler

© 2015 Hayle Medical

International Standard Book Number: 978-1-63241-375-8 (Hardback)

Printed in the United States of America.

Contents

Permissions

List of Contributors

Preface

Lack of well referenced, revised and standardized books on TB has led to formulation of this book sharing the clinical experiences of global professionals on TB. Data is being readily compiled from across the globe at a very fast rate about the efficiency of standardized treatment regimens for different forms of tuberculosis (TB) including drug-resistant TB, drug-sensitive TB and latent TB infection. At a time when we are facing the threat of multi drug-resistant TB [MDR-TB], development of extensively drug-resistant TB [XDR-TB] has threatened to undermine global efforts at TB control. This book covers in-depth analysis of all the developments and challenges in diagnosis and management of MDR-TB. Moreover, while physicians face the fatal disease of TB in their clinical practice, there have been several misunderstandings and controversies regarding various issues for the management and diagnosis of TB. The book covers topics like extra pulmonary tuberculosis and miscellaneous. Worldwide revival of MDR-TB shows that fight against this disease will continue in the coming years. The aim of this book is to serve as a valuable source of reference and guidance for the people who are involved in the management of TB as well as for the practicing physicians (especially, pulmonologists and internists).

This book unites the global concepts and researches in an organized manner for a comprehensive understanding of the subject. It is a ripe text for all researchers, students, scientists or anyone else who is interested in acquiring a better knowledge of this dynamic field.

I extend my sincere thanks to the contributors for such eloquent research chapters. Finally, I thank my family for being a source of support and help.

Editor

Extra Pulmonary Tuberculosis

Neurotuberculosis and HIV Infection

Simona Alexandra Iacob and Diana Gabriela Iacob

Additional information is available at the end of the chapter

1. Introduction

The incidence and mortality of tuberculosis (TB), the most common opportunistic infection in HIV patients has drastically increased with the emergence of the HIV pandemic

The HIV infection supported the re-emergence of TB as well as two major changes in the natural history of TB, namely it has increased the frequency of extrapulmonary TB and the mycobacterial multidrug resistance. The extrapulmonary TB involvement is present in up to 40% of the HIV cases and includes respiratory, digestive, lymphatic and neurologic localizations. Of these neurotuberculosis (NTB) is probably the most devastating extrapulmonary form of TB. The risk of acquiring NTB in HIV patients has been reported as 10 times higher than in non-HIV individuals and its related mortality exceeds 50%. The prognosis is further worsened by the HIV related progressive immunodeficiency which leads to the reactivation of opportunistic infections and the development of malignances. The early diagnosis of NTB in HIV positive patients improves the short and long term prognosis of these patients and increases their life expectancy. Unfortunately the complexity of the clinical presentation and the variability of the bacteriological results accounts for significant difficulties in the diagnostic confirmation of NTB. Therefore treatment in these patients is often empirical. Moreover the antituberculous treatment is of long duration with serious adverse effects. Ensuing complications during treatment include the immune reconstitution inflammatory syndrome (IRIS) - a complication that is characteristic for HIV patients undergoing treatment for TB. Furthermore the multiple drug interactions between the antituberculous and antiretroviral treatment require close supervision of these patients.

This chapter summarizes the epidemiological, pathogenic, clinic and therapeutic challenges of NTB in HIV patients.

This chapter summarizes the epidemiological, pathogenic, clinic and therapeutic challenges of NTB in HIV patients.

2. Epidemiological data on the HIV/TB co-infection

TB is preventable and curable and its eradication was considered possible before the spread of the HIV pandemic. Since then the pathogenic mechanisms of HIV and TB have been closely entwined. Such is the complementary evolution of HIV and TB that the HIV/TB co-infection has been referred to as a "syndemic" by some authors [1]. The term "syndemic" reflects the similar social, epidemiological and pathological settings of both diseases. The close interrelation between HIV and tuberculosis overcomes by far the interactions between other community acquired infections. Thus epidemiological studies suggest that as many as 50% of the HIV patients develop mycobacterial infections. The rate of extrapulmonary TB could account for more than 50% of cases presenting with HIV and TB coinfection. In the pre-AIDS era the immunodeficiency status incriminated in the pathogenesis of extrapulmonary TB was induced by autoimmune diseases, aging, diabetes, alcoholism, malnutrition, malignancies or immunosuppressive chemotherapy. However the total amount of extrapulmonary TB in non-HIV immunosupressed patients did not exceed 15% of all TB cases. In addition meningitis and other forms of NTB represented less than 1% of all TB cases in non-HIV patients [2,3] but presently account for 10% of all TB cases in HIV patients [4]. Tuberculous meningitis (TBM) occurs in 5%-8% of the HIV patients [5,6] but tuberculomas and abscesses are also a common finding in late stages of AIDS [7]. Regarding the CNS infection with non-tuberculous mycobacteria one of the most important risk factors is the progressive immunodeficiency induced by HIV infection.

Co-infection with HIV not only increases the risk for central nervous system (CNS) TB [17] but also alters the clinical signs, delays the diagnosis and worsens the prognosis [8]. Thus the mortality of HIV patients with TBM is as high as 63% and nearly half of deaths occur in the first 21 days [9].

3. Pathogenic mechanisms of NTB

TB is a respiratory infection with a generally latent course. The immunodeficiency status favors the extrapulmonary dissemination of mycobacteria leading to inflammatory granulomas with diverse localisations. Some granulomas arise adjacent to the meninges or to the brain parenchyma and become the last station before the CNS invasion. Disruption of these granulomas into the subarachnoid space is followed by the cerebrospinal fluid (CSF) invasion with mycobacteria and meningeal infection.Release of mycobacteria from these granulomas is mainly associated with the severe depletion of macrophages and lymphocytes along with the imbalance of local cytokines. The CSF inflammatory reaction induced by mycobacteria antigens leads to a lymphocyte and fibrin-rich subarachnoid exudate which progressively envelops the blood vessels and cranial nerves. The expansion and intensity of this inflammatory exudate induces multiple complications including: the obliterative vasculitis followed by cerebral infarctions, the CSF obstruction and emerging hydrocephalus and the spinal extension of TB and chronic arachnoiditis. Some of the CNS granulomas could evolve as cerebral or spinal masses further developing into tuberculomas or tuberculous abscesses [10,11,12]. In addition HIV patients characteristically present several TB cerebral lesions evolving simultaneously.

Below we enlisted the factors involved in the clinical progression and persistent CNS invasion with mycobacteria in HIV patients.

1. *The cellular immunosuppression in TB and HIV infection.*

    The site of extrapulmonary mycobacterial infections and especially the CNS invasion depend on the efficacy of cell-mediated immunity. Both the HIV infection and TB trigger complex mechanisms which increase the cellular immunosuppresion.

On the other hand humoral immnity is increased but inefficient. The high titres of antimycobacterial antibodies are not protective and could instead result in numerous complications. The most important mechanism behind the cellular immunosuppression in the HIV-TB coinfection is the severe depletion of macrophage and lymphocyte cells.

Macrophage and lymphocyte cells. Macrophages play a crucial role in both HIV and mycobacterial infections. As phagocytes of the innate immunity they are considered the main cells involved in the immune response against mycobacteria.Infected macrophages recruit additional immune cells such as dendritic cells and T cell lymphocytes and release numerous chemokines and cytokines to form granulomas. The latter are specific stable inflammatory structures limiting the growth of mycobacteria. At the same time mycobacteria could develop inside macrophages from granulomas thus ensuring their persistence. In addition macrophages infected with Mycobacterium tuberculosis (M. tbc) augment the expression of the C-C chemokine receptor type 5, also known as CCR5, the most important HIV coreceptor [13]. Therefore infected macrophages perform a significant role in the protection and transport of mycobacteria and HIV to other tissues including the brain.

With the passing of time some of the macrophages infected with mycobacteria suffer apoptosis leading to a numeric decrease of the most important cells involved in the defence against mycobacteria invasion. Moreover HIV is directly responsible for the depletion of CD4+ T lymphocytes through its cytopathic effect and anti-gp120 antibodies. The depletion of CD4+ T lymphocytes raises the susceptibility to TB and most notably towards neurologic forms of TB [14]. In this respect the decreasing CD4+ T cell count was proven to vary inversely with the incidence of NTB. Most patients with HIV and NTB display a CD4+ T cell count below 200 cells/ mm^3 unlike patients with pulmonary TB who commonly present with a CD4+T cell count, between 250 and 550 cells/ mm^3. In conclusion in the late stages of infection the main pathogenic mechanisms of invasion with mycobacteria and HIV are closely interwined.

The Cytokine dysregulation. Both HIV and mycobacteria are intracellular pathogens. Their presence stimulates the release of cytokines by macrophages and Th1 cells which in turn regulate the cells involved in the immune response. The stability of the granuloma is usually ensured by a high number of CD4+ T and CD8+ lymphocytes along with a Th1 cytokine profile represented by IFN -γ and TNF-α. [15].TNF-α is a pro-inflammatory cytokine released at high levels by CD4+T cells and macrophages coinfected with mycobacteria and HIV. The role of TNF-α in the clinical outcome of the 2 diseases is contradictory. Regarding its role in the control of tuberculosis a high level of TNF-α stimulates the apoptosis of infected macrophages and the cellular activation [16,17]. On the other hand the use of TNF-α neutralizing antibodies in inflammatory diseases has been associated with an increased risk of extrapulmonary TB including TBM [18].CD4-T-cell deficient mice [19] as well as mice able to neutralize endogenous TNf-α [20] or the gene for IFN-γ [21] are subjected to fatal TB. Nevertheless an in vitro experiment on human monocytes noted that higher levels of TNF-α could be associated with more virulent or faster growing mycobacterial strains [22].The contradictory effect of TNF-α was also observed in the HIV infection. Studies conducted by Lane and Osborn proved that TNF-α is a potent inhibitor over the primary HIV infection of the macrophages but enhances the HIV replication in latent HIV infections [23,24]. This finding could explain why mycobacteria infections which promote the synthesis of TNF-α could also augment HIV replication in chronic infected individuals. The level of TNF-α in the blood of patients infected with mycobacteria and HIV was documented to be 3 to 10 times higher than in non-HIV patients [25] showing a major imbalance in the release of this proinflammatory cytokine. TNF-α also plays a central role in the CNS localizations of mycobacteria. The excessive amount of TNF-α could accelerate the disruption of rich tuberculous foci adjacent to the CNS. Increased levels of TNF-α as well as IFN-γ were found in the CSF of patients with TBM at the disease onset [26] as well as several months after the acute episode [27] Experimental studies on rabbits proved that the excess of TNF-α acts as a persistent trigger of the inflammatory response and as a procoagulant factor associated with both the mycobacteria CNS invasion as well as cerebral vascular complications. [28]. The therapeutic use of TNF-α inhibitors in severe forms of TBM, tuberculoma and cerebral tuberculous abscesses was linked to a decreased inflammatory response and noticeable clinical recovery [29-31]. The major role of TNF-α in the progression of TBM was also proved in murine models by Tsenova as well [28,33]. Studies on HIV patients with TBM also emphasized the significance of increased levels of CSF TNF-α and of IFN-γ in advanced TBM stages [34].

In conclusion all these studies proved that important variations of the Th1 cytokine profile and especially of those involving the release of TNF-α represent one of the pathogenic mechanisms that aggravate the outcome of NTB in the HIV infection. Understanding these changes could be the first step towards the development of efficient complementary therapies in NTB to reduce the excessive inflammatory response. Thus TNF-α inhibition could be used as an antiinflammatory therapy in NTB with severe complications but should not be recommended in other forms of TB.

2.   *The persistent activation of microglial cells.*

A significant role in the pathogenic mechanisms of CNS infections was assigned to the activation of microglial cells, the resident macrophages of the CNS. Microglial cells are involved in the local phagocytosis and play a central role in the pathogenesis of infections and inflammatory diseases [35]. These cells also represent the main target of both HIV and mycobacteria infection [36,37]. Thus the activation of microglial cells by mycobacteria induces the release of proinflammatory cytokines, some of which are able to add to the stability of cerebral granulomas. A moderate level of CXCL9 and CXCL10 chemokines released by microglial cells regulates the influx of inflammatory cells to the brain and interferes with the chemotaxis of monocytes/macrophages and T cells thus assisting the formation of granulomas. However since microglial cells are the main source of cerebral TNF-α these could also induce an aggresive inflammatory response with severe meningeal inflammation, brain edema, protein accumulation, endarteritis and intracranial hypertension accounting for most of the complications described in NTB [28,38]. Therefore a balanced activation of microglial cells is critical against the CNS mycobacterial invasion. On the other hand the intracellular HIV replication in microglial cells leads to their activation, neuroinflammation and release of neurotoxins that cause AIDS associated neural dysfunctions. The complex role of the microglia in cerebral HIV/TB co-infection is explained by the rich number of HIV receptors and co-receptors expressed by these cells such as CD4, CCR5, CXCR4 as well as other receptors involved in the inflammatory response including IFN-γ, TNF-α,CD14 and MHC class I and II receptors [39].The CD14 receptor promotes the uptake of both HIV and nonopsonized M.tbc strains in microglial cells [40] while CD4 and CCR5/CXCR4 co-receptors interfere with HIV cell attachment. As a result microgial cells are the main target of HIV and mycobacteria once these enter the CNS. Therapies directed towards reducing the inflammatory response in the HIV/TB co-infection include the blockage of certain receptors (such as CD14), the use of CCR5 antagonists and TNF-α blockers (as thalidomide). Another alternative is dexametasone recommended in most forms of CNS TB. The clinical benefits of dexametazone were inspired by in vitro studies proving a potent inhibitory effect on the release of cytokines from microglia [39].

In conclusion simultaneous infection of the microglia with HIV and mycobacteria increases the meningeal inflammatory response, the fundamental pathogenic step in all forms of CNS TB. The synthesis of excessive inflammatory infiltrate is responsible for the clinical findings and possibly irreversible complications in NTB, such as hydrocephalus and vasculitis [41]. Moreover the excessive inflammatory response triggered in the HIV/TB co-infection could induce the immune reconstitution inflammatory syndrome – a complication that is specific for this patient category.

4. Pathogenesis of the immune reconstitution inflammatory syndrome

The Immune Reconstitution Inflammatory Syndrome (IRIS) is an uncommon inflammatory response encountered in those cases of severe immunosuppression in which the rapid administration of specific treatment abruptly restores the immune response. The HIV infection is the most frequent cause of immunodeficiency predisposing to IRIS. In addition TB is the most common opportunistic infection related to HIV-associated IRIS. The antiretroviral and antituberculous treatments rapidly restore the immune response. Such a rapid treatment response may sometimes lead to an aggressive lymphoproliferative reaction and massive release of proinflammatory cytokines. There are 2 clinical presentations of IRIS known as the paradoxical IRIS and unmasking IRIS. IRIS manifestations in HIV patients with NTB follow two possible scenarios:

a. A paradoxical reaction emerging in patients with NTB correctly diagnosed and appro-
    priately treated in which HIV infection is subsequently detected and also treated but new
    severe neurological manifestations arise during treatment (paradoxical NeuroIRIS-TB).

b. An unmasking reaction appears in patients with HIV and latent unknown NTB in which
    the successful antiretroviral treatment unexpectedly induces neurological manifestations
    of TB (unmasked NeuroIRIS-TB)

The neurologic manifestation of IRIS-TB are rare (19% of the total cases) but with a mortality risk
that is three times higher than other IRIS localisations [42]. The specific features related to
NeuroIRIS-TB reside in the excessive CNS inflammatory reactions generated by the activation
of microglia. The excessive inflammatory response is linked to the abundance of mycobacterial antigens and their high immunogenicity. Various studies have approached the immunologic mechanisms and risk factors for IRIS in HIV-TB patients.

The observations below on the pathogenesis of IRIS-TB were selected according to the potential
clinical application.

• The release of multiple mycobacterial antigens in the first 2 months of antituberculous
  therapy and concurrent wide distribution of sequestered CD45RO memory lymphocytes in
  the bloodstream during HIV antiretroviral treatment are the principal mechanisms inducing
  an excessive inflammatory response. To avoid the overlap of these events the current WHO
  recommendations advocate an initial antituberculous treatment followed at a minimum
  interval of 2 weeks by the antiretroviral treatment in patients with a low level of Th CD4+
  cells [43]

• The pathological overproduction of Th1 cytokines particularly IFN-γ was noticed in IRIS-
  TB/ HIV co-infection [44,45].Taking into account the experimentally increased levels of IFN-
  γ in IRIS the blood interferon-gamma (IFN-γ) release assays (IGRA) could be implemented
  to monitor IRIS evolution in the future. In addition the pathological overproduction of
  chemokines CXCL9 and CXCL10 induced by IFN-γ was observed in IRIS-TB/HIV co-
  infection [46]. The development of therapeutic strategies which could reduce the intracerebral level of these chemokines are essential to prevent and decrease ensuing granulomas
  thus protecting against IRIS.[47,48]

• The excessive release of IgG antibodies to PPD was observed in patients with IRIS-TB/HIV
  co-infection [45] Nonetheless the level of antibodies against the phenolic glycolipid antigen
  (PGL-TB1) was lower in IRIS hosts. The IgG anti PPD and especially the intrathecal synthesis
  of IgG/PPD could provide additional information on the humoral immune response in
  NeuroIRIS – TB [49].

• The restoration of a delayed type of hypersensitivity to mycobacterial antigens was reported
  in HIV patients with latent TB after starting the antiretroviral therapy [50,51]. All the same
  recent studies cast doubt on the tuberculin-specific Th1-responses in prompting IRIS [52]

• The profile of cytokines differs between the 2 types of IRIS as well as between TB infection
  and IRIS-TB. Hence certain cytokines (IFN-γ,TNF-α and IL-6) are more elevated in IRIS-TB
  than compared with patients presenting only TB. [53,54]. This finding could help distinguish

TB from IRIS-TB. Other studies have also investigated different profiles of immunological markers which could aid in the above distinction. Conradie et al. have identified a profile of makers including IL8, active NK cells, C reactive protein and lymphocyte count that is related to unmasking IRIS-TB. This profile could be further used in the differential diagnosis of the 2 manifestations or as a prediction of unmasking IRIS-TB [55].

5. Etiological data on the mycobacterial strains in HIV/TB co-infection

HIV patients are frequently infected by virulent strains of M.tbc. The virulence of a particular strain depends on the genetic composition of M.tbc. Thus the Beijing genotype of M.tbc mostly found in Asia is considered the most aggressive genotype and has been associated with CSF dissemination and multidrug resistance to antituberculous agents in HIV patients [56]. Infections with M. bovis are rare and occur mostly in HIV Hispanic patients. Despite the high environmental exposure to nontuberculous mycobacteria CNS involvement is rare even in AIDS patients and usually occurs at a CD4+ count under 10 cells/mm3. The pathogenic mechanisms behind the interactions established between the host and virulent mycobacteria are less documented. The infection with Mycobacterium avium complex (MAC) remains the most studied and most frequent nontuberculous mycobacteria accounting for the atypical tuberculous manifestations in the advanced stages of AIDS infection [57]. The Mycobacterium avium intracellulare (MAI) serotypes 4 and 8 are the most prevalent in AIDS patients [58].

Sporadic cases of NTB with other mycobacteria have also been recorded in AIDS patients following disseminated infection [59]. MAC is an ubiquitary environmental mycobacteria which colonizes the gastrointestinal and respiratory tract but is also able to invade the epithelial cells and the intestinal wall [60]. Virulent strains isolated from AIDS patients are able to penetrate the mucosal barriers and resist intracellular killing by macrophages resulting in a disseminated infection. Further studies on the interaction between M. avium and the HIV-infected cells confirmed the inhibition of several cytokines secreted by the Th_1 CD4+cells, natural killer cells and macrophages.These ultimately favour the intracellular survival of M. avium and even accelerate its growth rate [61,62]. The neurologic involvement due to MAC in advanced stages of AIDS generally presents as TBM following a disseminated infection with prolonged bacteremia [63-66]. The comparative aspects of the CNS invasions with M.tbc and nontuberculous mycobacteria in HIV hosts are presented in table 1

6. Clinical data on NTB in HIV patients

NTB is frequent in HIV patients compared with non-HIV patients. Reactivation of latent forms of TB is accelerated in HIV patients with a 10% annual risk of progression to active infection compared with 10-20% lifetime risk of developing TB in non-HIV patients. Literature data is contradictory as to the role of HIV on the clinical presentation or evolution of NTB. Although some studies found significant differences between HIV and non-HIV NTB [67-69] others

	M. tbc	Nontuberculous mycobacteria
Mycobacteria strain	M tbc, rarely M bovis	98% MAC, rarely other mycobacteria
Primary infection	Usually respiratory	Gastrointestinal or respiratory
Frequency	Moderate	Low/very low
CD4+ T cell count	< 200 cells/mm3	<10% cells/mm3 (usually)
Clinical forms	Meningitis, Tuberculoma, Abscess	Disseminated, Abscess
Diagnosis	Established diagnosis criteria	No standard diagnosis criteria
CSF mycobacteria detection	Essential to diagnosis confirmation	Not essential to diagnosis confirmation
Mycobacteria detection (other than CSF)	In blood	In faeces (frequently), in blood (if disseminated infections)
Prognosis	Reserved	Terminal infections (frequently)

Table 1. Comparative aspects of the CNS invasions with M. tbc and nontuberculous mycobacteria in HIV hosts

argued that the HIV co-infection does not influence the clinical evolution [70]. Nevertheless the differential diagnosis between NTB and numerous systemic and neurologic nontuberculous complications emerging in AIDS is difficult. Thus the clinical presentation of NTB in HIV patients could be influenced by numerous factors such as:

- various neurological manifestations caused by HIV itself;
- other opportunistic infections with CNS tropism, mainly toxoplasma, criptococcus, papilloma or herpes viruses infections;
- concurrent cerebral tumors : non-Hodkin cerebral lymphoma, Kaposi sarcoma;
- simultaneous evolution of various forms of NTB (meningitis, tuberculoma)- a characteristic finding in HIV patients;
- extra-neurological infections or malignancies related to HIV.

All these interfering factors could explain the variable descriptions of the clinical presentation, CSF manifestations or imaging aspects in the numerous studies on NTB in HIV patients.

NTB in HIV patients encompasses the following forms: TBM, disseminated TB of the nevrax, tuberculoma, and tuberculous abcess. En plaque tuberculoma, chronic spinal pahymeningitis and serous TBM are rare forms of TB not described in HIV patients.

6.1. Tuberculous meningitis in HIV patients

The real frequency of TBM in HIV patients is hard to assess as the various clinical presentations related to immunodepression could be confused with other neurologic manifestations. The epidemiological data on the subject is contradictory. Current statistics in areas with an increased prevalence of TB disclose M. tbc as the most frequent etiologic agent of meningitis in HIV patients [71]. Moreover TBM was recorded as the initial presentation of AIDS in 42% of cases. A study performed in Kenya, a state with an increasing incidence of TB and HIV, revealed that 80% of the necropsies performed on HIV patients exhibited disseminated TB and 26% of these also displayed meningeal involvement [72].On the other hand the frequency of disseminated tuberculosis based on clinical and bacteriological criteria only did not exceed 14,5% of cases [73-74]. The conclusion arising from these studies is that the extent of the CNS invasion is highly variable and a large number of disseminated TB in AIDS probably remains undiagnosed.

Neurological presentation. TBM is the most frequent form of NTB in HIV patients. The neurological manifestations differ according to the degree of immunodeficiency.

- *TBM in the early stages of HIV immunodepression.* The onset of TBM is insidious. Fever and meningeal signs develop progressively (7-30 days) paralleling the changes in the cognitive status and mental state. Once the meningeal syndrome is established the evolution is rapid. The meningeal syndrome is intense and progressive. Under such circumstances the diagnosis could be aided by recognizing the paralysis of certain cranial nerves (mostly involving the sixth cranial nerve but also the second, third, fourth and eighth nerves) as well as the signs of hydrocephalus or cerebral edema (headache, convulsions, pyramidal or cerebellar signs). Encephalitic forms display an altered level of consciousness with progressive evolution to coma. In forms with major spinal involvement (TB spinal meningitis, spinal arachnoiditis) the inflammatory exudate surrounds the spinal cord and induces radicular compression. As a result radicular pains develop along with sings of transverse mielitis (paraplegia and urine retention).

- *TBM in advanced stage of HIV immunodepression.* In advanced stage of immunodepression the inflammatory exudate is decreased and the clinical presentation is atypical. Fever could be absent in these patients. The meningeal sings are discrete or missing [75]. Hydrocephalus is delayed. Tuberculous vasculopathy prompts frequent complications following thrombosis, or hemorrhagic infarcts. Focal lesions related to the vasculopathy are common. The cognitive dysfunction is severe [76] with a rapid evolution to profound coma [8].In this advanced stage of AIDS NTB rarely evolves as a solitary finding. Usually other infections or tumors are also associated with NTB and the wide spectrum of clinical manifestations implies various *neurological patterns with focal, perypheral or central nervous signs.*

CSF data. The aspect of the initial CSF could be suggestive disclosing lymphocytic pleocytosis, elevated proteins and low glucose levels. Nevertheless the etiologic confirmation is based on bacteriological criteria only. In patients with severe immunodeficiency the CSF white cell count is usually only slightly increased but could also be normal [67] The low number of lymphocytes in HIV could modify the differential count in the CSF to a predominant number of neutrophils [67] causing confusion with bacterial meningitis. Elevated proteins are a typical finding in TBM in non-HIV patients. However 43% of the HIV reported cases presented low or even normal protein values [5,8]. The most difficult cases are those in which the CSF is reported as normal, a common finding in patients with severe immunodeficiency. In the absence of a strong inflammatory response acid-fast bacilli smear retrieves positive results [67] in up to 67% of cases and the cultures are positive in 40 – 87,9% of cases [76,77].High rates of smear and culture positivity facilitate the diagnosis in patients with an atypical clinical presentation and normal CSF exam.

Neuroradiological findings. The classic CT neuroradiological findings in TBM include basal meningeal enhancement, hydrocephalus, and infarctions in the supratentorial brain parenchyma and brainstem [78]. The concurrent finding of basal meningeal enhancement, tuberculoma or both on CT scans could disclose a sensitivity of 89% and 100% specificity for TBM in non-HIV patients [79]. In HIV patients contrast-enhanced MRI is generally considered superior to CT results [78]. Some MRI studies indicated that meningeal enhancement and cerebral infarctions were more common in HIV-infected individuals with TBM by comparison with non-HIV patients [5,70]. However the basal meningeal enhancement and hydrocephalus rarely occur in advanced stages of AIDS with reduced inflammatory response [76]. On the other hand cerebral infarctions and focal mass lesions are frequently encountered in late stages of AIDS [80-82]. In addition to the previous aspects imaging studies also disclose cerebral atrophy due to HIV infection. Tubeculomas also were reported in 15-24% of cases [5].

6.1.1. The diagnosis of TBM in HIV infected patients

The diagnosis is urgent and extensive including all tuberculous lesions, HIV status and other HIV associated lesions, bacteriological confirmation and neurological complications. It is based on clinical features, CSF analysis and MRI imaging. (table 2). A belated diagnosis increases the mortality, complications and the risk of relapse.

Clinical diagnostic criteria. Clinical features in HIV patients with TBM reflect the atypical inflammatory response and the extensive vasculopathy. The meningeal sings are inconstant and discrete especially in patients with severe immunodepression. The signs of encephalitis emerge from the onset and could be the first significant manifestation of the disease. The gravity of the altered level of consciousness parallels the increased mortality [8].Cerebral nerve paralysis is a common finding but could be also induced by other associated conditions such as HIV neurotoxicity, the cerebral reactivation of opportunistic infections (toxoplasma, JS virus, Herpes simplex virus) or cerebral malignancies (Non-Hodgkin lymphoma, Kaposi sarcoma). These patients particularly exhibit multiple extraneurologic manifestations. The presence of other active lesions like pulmonary TB or other extrameningeal sites of TB is highly suggestive for the CNS TB diagnosis [5,67,81]. Thus the presentation of HIV patients unlike non-HIV patients often includes peripheral, intrathoracic and intraabdominal adenopathies. The etiology of these adenopathies does not always imply a diagnosis of TB. The differential diagnosis for adenopathies should always include other lymphotropic opportunistic infections with neurologic manifestations (toxoplasma, CMV, syphilis). The tuberculous origin of adenopathies could be overestimated in the clinical diagnosis if the histological confirmation is not obtained. The histological examination is thus a prerequisite for a correct diagnosis of these adenopathies. Hepatosplenomegaly is commonly reported but could also occur as a result of other HIV associated infections (B or C hepatitis, CMV infections).To conclude no clinical criteria is highly suggestive for CNS TB in HIV patients. Moreover any neurologic or extraneurologic finding should prompt a thorough differential diagnosis that includes any other HIV related affections.

Laboratory diagnostic criteria. The degree of immunodeficiency in HIV patients with NTB could be assessed using the CD4+T cell count. Most studies on TBM disclose a CD4+T cell count between 32-200 /mm^3 [5,81,82].Other findings including a lower hematocrit, peripheral low neutrophils, lower plasma sodium level [76] and moderate to severe anemia Hb < 8 gm/dl [69] were not constantly present in all studies and could be mostly related to the HIV infection than to TB. Moreover hyponatremia in patients with HIV-TB co-infection could arise due to the following: a) cerebral salt wasting syndrome observed in 65% of patients with numerous cerebral lesions, including patients with TBM [83]; b) the syndrome of inappropriate release of antidiuretic hormone secretion; c) hypothalamus pituitary-adrenal axis suppresion. Hyponatremia is a marker of the disease severity and the mortality in this patient group is significantly higher than that of patients with normal sodium levels (36,5% versus 19.7%) [84].

The CSF exam is decisive for the diagnosis. The specificity of the bacteriological diagnosis is 100% but its implication in the final diagnosis is quite low since the Ziehl-Neelsen stain is positive in less than 20% of cases and Lowenstein culture confirmation although positive in 73% of cases is tardy [85]. Methods of improving the sensibility of Ziehl-Neelsen stain have been described [86] but are less implemented. Tuberculin skin test and Interferon-gamma release assays if positive do not distinguish between latent TB and active disease. As well negative results should be evaluated with caution in severely immunodepressed patients. Several complementary diagnostic tools were explored in certain studies like specific antigens and antibodies detection, adenosine deaminase detection, PCR techniques, detection of tuberculostearic acid or IFN-γ levels in the CSF. However their use is limited due to discordant results or other inconveniences related to the cost, cross-reactivity, specificity or sensibility [87-90]. Recently the improvement of nucleic acid amplification assay techniques, particularly polymerase chain reaction (PCR) assay (especially nested PCR assay technique) increased the diagnostic sensitivity and specificity but its use in AIDS related CNS TB is still unconfirmed [91]. All in all the bacteriological confirmation is difficult and belated but remains the only diagnostic tool in AIDS related CNS TB.

Imaging diagnostic criteria. Imaging studies are required in the evaluation of neurological complications of TBM, in the treatment follow-up and differential diagnosis. Contrast enhanced MRI and Positron emission computed tomography – computed tomography (PET-CT) display the highest sensibility. Unfortunately most literature studies are based on the more inexpensive CT scans. No aspects are definitely characteristic to CNS TB in HIV patients. Atypical results showing the absence or minimal meningeal enhancement [8] or the absence of communicating hydrocephalus were reported on the CT scan in 69% of AIDS cases [5,8]. Nevertheless other studies found no significant radiological differences between HIV and non-HIV patients.

*In addition to the clinical, CSF and radiologic criteria, a medical history of TB and positive tuberculin skin test could help raise the diagnostic suspicion of a tuberculous infection.

Neurotuberculosis suspicion
Clinical investigations (assessing the risk of tuberculosis, neurological manifestations, other manifestations)
History of tuberculosis (TB antecedents, risk of exposure)
Physical examination disclosing:
1. Signs of menigeal irritation (suggesting meningitis or a meningeal reaction to localized cerebral lesions)
2. Neurologic examination (mental status, sensory and motor exam, focal signs, intracranial hypertension)
3. Other manifestations suggesting TB and nontuberculous lesions induced by HIV activity, opportunistic infections or malignancies like lymphadenopathy (given attention to lymphoma, syphilis, toxoplasmosis), pleural or pericardial effusion (given attention to Kaposi sarcoma), pulmonary lesion (given attention to pneumocystosis, Kaposi sarcoma, fungal pneumonia,CMV pneumonia, lymphocytic interstitial pneumonitis), skin lesions (given attention to Kaposi sarcoma, Moluscum contagiosum, fungal lesions, meningococcal purpura)
Laboratory data assessing the immune status, HIV activity, risk of opportunistic infections or malignancies
Complete blood count (pancytopenia suggests medullar invasion with mycobacteria but also invasive malignancies or drug toxicities)
Biochemical evaluation of liver and renal function; indicate associated co-morbidities; important for drug regimen recomandation,
Serum sodium level (hyponatremia is linked to disseminated mycobacteriosis and cerebral lesions/ it corelates with the mortality risk)
Immune status: CD4+ T cell count (CD4<200 cells/mm^3 is related to the risk of NTB and major HIV-related opportunistic infections; CD4< 50 cells/mm^3 is related to the risk of nontuberculous mycobacteriosis or to the risk of IRIS)
HIV viral status: blood/CSF RNA HIV viral load (if positive it point to the antiretroviral failure and needing to swich the regimen)
Serologic assays: serum specific antibodies IgG and IgM related to other HIV-opportunistic infections,mainly toxoplasma, CMV, syphilis.
Imaging studies: cerebral or spinal CT/MRI; (important in localized NTB and other cerebral opportunistic infections or malignancies
Eye fundus examination : shows choroid tubercles in disseminated tuberculosis
Neurotuberculosis confirmation
Lumbar puncture (if the MRI does not indicate mass lesions!): CSF analysis: cytochemistry, stains*, culture **, or complementary exams ***!
Other specimens analysis: sputum, pleural fluid, blood, urine, tissue specimens (lymph node, hepatic or cerebral biopsy): stains*, culture** other examination***

, human immunodeficiency virus; CSF, cerebrospinal fluid; TB, tuberculosis; NTB, neurotuberculosis; MRI, magnetic resonance imaging;CMV, citomegalvirus; * stains: Ziehl Neelsen (acid-fast bacilli), India ink (fungi), Gram smear (bacteria); ** culture on specific media: Lowestein or Bactec(mycobacteria), Sabourraud (fungi), blood agar (bacteria); *** PCR,polymerase chain reaction, detection of ADA activity, detection of antigens/ antibodies for toxoplasma, CMV, criptococcus, meningococcus, pneumococcus

Table 2. Neurotuberculosis diagnosis in HIV patients

6.1.2. The evolution of TBM in HIV patients

In the HIV-TB co-infection TBM is frequently associated with pulmonary TB or tuberculous lymphadenopathies. *The risk of a relapse* is considered 23%. The most important risk of relapse is the lack of adherence to the antituberculous and antiretroviral treatment. CSF blood glucose ratio and the presence of pulmonary TB could also be linked with the risk of relapse according to a study performed in Vietnam [92]. *The mortality rate* is high; the survival rate is difficult to evaluate taking into account the increased mortality of HIV patients due to other opportunistic infections or specific complications. Risk factors for death during hospitalization for TBM included: a) the CD4+ count lower than 50 cells/mm^3; b) the presence of advanced neurologic signs or hydrocephalus on admission; c) a diagnosis and treatment delay with more than 3 days [80];d) the absence of the antiretroviral treatment or failure of the highly active antiretroviral therapy (HAART) [93].TBM relapsing forms and multidrug resistant mycobacteria are linked to a high mortality rate. IRIS prognosis is generally good.

6.1.3. Conclusion

TBM comprises variable manifestations in HIV patients. Early stages of immunodepression in HIV patients usually set the same diagnostic difficulties as in non-HIV patients as a result of the variable clinical presentations and delayed bacteriological results. In the advanced stages of HIV the clinical presentation is atypical and the CSF cytochemical profile could be within normal parameters. Other concurrent lesions of active TB could ease the diagnosis. The differential diagnosis should always include other HIV-associated manifestations, other opportunistic infections or malignancies. The bacteriological exam is still the only tool able to confirm the diagnosis. The prognosis of TBM in HIV patients is shadowed by numerous diagnostic difficulties, increased risk of relapse and associated HIV pathology.

Below are NTB diagnosis criteria (table 2) and imaging aspects found in our clinical practice in patients with HIV and NTB: meningoencephalitis (figure 1), cerebral tuberculoma (figure 2) and cerebral tuberculoma in context of IRIS (figure 3)

6.2. CNS disseminated TB

CNS disseminated TB (CNS milliary TB, cerebrospinal granulia) is a form of cerebral milliary frequently associated with disseminated TB. It is rarely limited to the CNS. The diagnosis is usually based on findings at the necropsy or MRI results. *Constitutional symptoms develop progressively even in the absence of neurologic signs; mycobacteria could also be isolated in other pathological products than the CSF (most frequently from the blood). The eye fundus exam could disclose characteristic choroid tubercles.* A classical miliary pattern on chest radiograph frequently complements the aspects of cerebral miliary. Postconstrast MR brain images reveal intense nodular enhancing granulomas located at cortico-medulary junction and throughout the brain parenchyma. The differential diagnosis of cerebral military should include other opportunistic disseminated infections or secondary metastatic lesions. It is possible to underestimate this form of CNS TB as a result of the diagnostic difficulties and required expensive imaging studies.

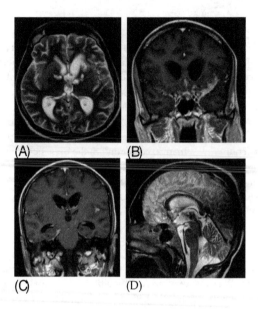

Figure 1. A-D. Cranio-cerebral MR: axial (A), coronal (B and C), and saggital (D) images showing tuberculous meningi-tis, cerebral thrombosis and hidrocephalus in a 23-year-old patient with AIDS. He had been receiving antiretroviral treatment for 3 months prior to the present hospitalization. He was admitted with milliary TB and meningoencephalitis associated with oral HCV infection, candidiosis and reactivated CMV infection. The clinical evolution was complicated by toxic hepatitis due to antituberculous treatment and cerebral thrombosis. On admission the CD4 count was 244/mm^3 and the RNA HIV load was 239 copies/ml. Contrast MRI before and after the administration of intravenous gadolinium and angioMRI(sag 3D PC phlebography) show: hyperintense lesions on FLAIR sequences and T2 weighted images, appearing hypointense on T1 with no contrast enhancement, located in the medial part of the lentiform nucleus and the head of the caudate nucleus; contrast filling of the basal cisterns extending to the sylvian fissure (more proeminent on the left side), the floor of the third ventricule and the infundibular area (involving the optic nerves, chiasm and optic tracts); asymmetric profound venous system with bilateral amputation of the superios talamostriate veins without the visualisation of the anterior left vein of the pellucid septum; enlargement of the ventricular system with no median shift or transependimar resorbtion. *Conclusions:* post ischemic sequelae, thrombosis of the profound venous system, basal meningeal contrast enhance-ment suggestive for meningitis and dilation of the ventricular system.

6.3. Intracranial mass lesions in HIV patients with CNS TB

6.3.1. Tuberculoma

CNS tuberculomas develop insidiously in the cerebral parenchyma following either the reactivation of local granulomas [94] or a paradoxical response to the antituberculous therapy (figure 2,3). The lesions could be solitary or multiple and their localisations are diverse. Cerebral localisations are more frequent than spinal ones. Data on HIV patients presenting tuberculomas is scarce [95,96]. The diagnosis is probably underestimated in low income countries taking into account the expensive CT/MRI importance in the confirmation. The clinical presentation is pseudotumoral with fever and headaches. The neurologic signs vary according to localisation and may be absent. HIV patients rarely present signs of intracranial hypertension or convulsions. On the other hand tuberculomas could be associated with other

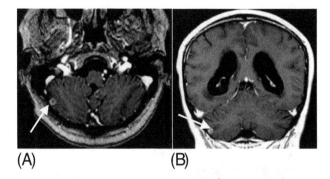

(A)   (B)

Figure 2. Cranio-cerebral *MR images* showing cerebelous tuberculoma in a 41 year-old patient with a 5 year history of HIV infection nonadherent to the antiretroviral treatment.The patient was admitted with a cerebellous tuberculoma and acute ischemic stroke.The laboratory data on admission disclosed a CD4 count of 145cells/mm³ and RNA HIV load 240000 copies/ml.*Axial T1 weighted images shows (A)*: Focal enchancing triangular lesion in the anterolateral right-side of the pons of 5x9 mm with FLAIR hyperintensity, difussion restriction, no significant changes in the apparent diffusion coefficient (ADC) and no contrast enhancement (the aspect is suggestive for acute ischemia); a right focal cortico-subcortical cerebellous lesion with peripheral ring enhancement on T1 weighted images and mass effect (the aspect is compatible with a tuberculoma). *Coronal T1 weighted images shows (B)*: symmetrical enlargement of the ventricular system with no midline shift; transependimar circumferential resorbtion edema is present adjacent to the ventricular wall; no intraventricular obstruction or contrast enhancement. *Conclusions*: acute ischemic stroke in the anterolateral right side of the pons; focalinferolateral parenchymal lesion suggestive for a tuberculoma; significant hydrocephalus with no intraventricular obstruction.

manifestations of TB such as TBM, pulmonary TB or other signs suggestive for CNS TB such as tuberculous vasculitis. The CSF usually displays no changes or few cytochemical abnormal findings (low glucose, elevated proteins); the acid-fast bacilli smear and culture are frequently negative. The aspect on the CT suggestive for a tuberculoma presents as isodense or lightly hypodense lesions with annular contrast enhancement and the "target sign" as a result of central calcifications. Nevertheless these aspects are not pathognomonic and the diagnosis requires a cerebral biopsy with histological and bacteriological confirmation. The histopathological examination usually discloses a central region of caseous necrosis surrounded by a capsule with a granulomatous structure. This aspect evolves dynamically as follows: 1) noncaseating granuloma; 2) caseating granuloma with a solid center; 3) caseating granuloma with a liquid center. This dynamics could also be detected at the contrast enhanced MRI or MRI spectroscopy as opposed to the images induced by a cerebral abscess. The MRI examination indicates a correspondent evolution with the histopatological examination as: 1) hypointense lesions on T1-weighted images (T1W) and hyperintense T2W lesions with nodular enhancemen postgadolinium administration; 2) hypointense lesions on T1W and T2W with peripheral rim enhancement postgadolinium ;3) hypointense T1W and hyperintense T2W with hypointense rim postgadolinium. Difussion weigthed images indicate diffusion restriction within the tuberculoma. The lesions are surrounded by edema. The lesions in HIV patients often appear as ring-enhancement lesions under 1 cm and the mass effect is rarely seen [97]. The CT/MRI aspect should be distinguished from other ring-enhancing lesions including bacterial cerebral abscesses, cerebral toxoplasmosis, CNS cryptococcosis, neurocysticercosis or CNS lymphomas.

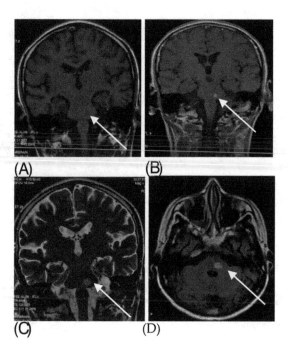

Figure 3. Cranio-cerebral *MRI*, showing left pontine tuberculoma in a 16 year-old patient previously diagnosed and undergoing treated for lymph node TB for the past 2 months and recently diagnosed with HIV infection.The patient also associated HBV and CMV infection and oral candidiosis.On admission the patient was in coma. The laboratory data displayed a CD4 count of 24 cells/mm³ and RNA HIV 1064973copies/ml. Final diagnosis was NeuroIRIS TB (tuberculoma).The CSF disclosed no changes.The clinical evolution was favourable. *A:* coronal T_1 weighted image demonstrating left pontine paramedian nodular lesion of 4 mm surrounded by perilesional edema (discrete hyposignal). *B:* coronal section T_1 postcontrast shows hypersignal; C- coronal section T_2 and D- axial FLAIR section show intense contrast uptake and no diffusion restriction.

6.3.2.Tuberculous abscess

The tuberculous abscess represents a purulent collection delineated by a capsule with a granulomatous structure. This is a rare finding in immunocompetent patients as well as in the early stages of AIDS but common in severe immunodeficiency states with CD4+T cell count under 100/mm³ [96]. The tuberculous abscess results from the liquefaction of tuberculomas [13] or from the necrotic evolution of granulomas in the setting of severe immunodeficiency [98].The necrotic centre is invaded by mycobacteria. The CSF is unchanged. The evolution is more acute than tuberculomas with neurologic deficit, fever and headaches [96, 99-100]. The CT/MRI aspect resembles the images in caseous tuberculomas but the lesion is larger (>3cm), multilobulated, surrounded by a thick capsule and ring enhancement. The perilesional edema and the mass effect are the most important features. The histological and bacteriological exam the cerebral biopsy confirm the diagnosis. The differential diagnosis includes other intracranial space-occupying lesions especially cerebral toxoplasmosis and lymphoma [19].In such cases PCR techniques could increase the diagnostic yield [101,102].

7. Infections with non-tuberculous mycobacteria in HIV patients

Nontuberculous mycobacteria induce CNS lesions especially in AIDS patients with advanced stages of immunodepression. Sporadic cases triggered by M. avium, M. kanssasi, M. fortuitum, M gordonae, M. genavense and M. terrae were reported [105,106]. As a rule CNS infections with non-tuberculous mycobacteria are the result of MAC infection. Nevertheless infection with MAC shows no predilection for the CNS as it frequently colonises the respiratory and gastrointestinal tract. Disseminated infections occur as a result of a severe immune dysfunction at a CD4 count under 60 cells/mm^3 [57]. Under 10 cells/ mm^3 the neurological dissemination is also possible [107]. However a case study reported by Fletcher disclosed a cerebral abscess with a double etiology involving M tbc and MAC in an AIDS patient with a CD+4 count of 140 cells/mm^3 [108]. Higher values of the CD4+ count were also found in cases of MAC–related IRIS in the absence of a systemic infection [109]. Most MAC neurologic manifestations in HIV infected patients are cerebral abscesses and meningoencephalitis. Localized mass lesions (including single or multiple abscesses) contain a large number of mycobacteria in the absence of the typical granulomatous structure. These findings are frequently accompanied by pleocytosis and an occasionally high protein level on CSF examination. The diagnosis should be confirmed by a histological exam (in cerebral localized forms) or by using minimum 2 hemocultures (in disseminated forms). MAC was also isolated in the CSF in disseminated forms. NeuroIRIS-MAC associated manifestations were sporadically reported in HIV patients [110].

8. The treatment of NTB in HIV patients

The treatment of NTB in HIV patients should be combined, controlled and individualized.

1. The antituberculous and antiretroviral medication must be *combined* according to the synergistic drug interactions; the doses in the combined scheme must be adjusted to prevent treatment resistance.

2. The drug regimen must be *controlled* for adherence, drug interactions, toxicities, clinical response and treatment resistance

3. Treatment must be *individualized* and adapted to other co-morbidities, associated therapies and hypersensitivity reactions of the patient

The main antituberculous and antiretroviral classes, their corresponding representative drugs, pharmacological interactions, adverse reactions and treatment efficacy are shown in table 3. The NTB treatment principles in HIV patients are presented in accordance with the European AIDS Clinical Society guidelines, CDC and American Thoracic Society recomandations [111-113].

8.1. The antituberculous treatment

Treatment of tuberculous meningitis. TBM is a curable disease. Response to treatment in patients with NTB and HIV is similar to patients diagnosed with TB only. The elevated mortality is a result of the belated diagnosis, resistant mycobacteria and severe immunodeficiency

- **The main characteristics of the antituberculous treatment in HIV patients with NTB**

1. Treatment should be urgently started based on clinical and biological data, CSF modifications, the history of TB, other tuberculous lesions and imaging studies. The CSF specimens should be collected for culture and for resistance detection before treatment starting. The bacteriological confirmation should not delay the treatment as the treatment delay accounts for a poor prognosis. Advanced stages of the disease with irreversible complications (hydrocephalia, adherences, cerebral infarcts) are related to high mortality rates.

2. The antituberculous therapy must have increased CSF penetration (table 3) [114-120].

3. Corticosteroid therapy should be initiated as early as possible and continued for 6–8 weeks.

4. A long course of therapy for a minimum of 12 months is strong recomended.

- **Factors to consider**

1. *Combined treatment* must include an *initial phase* of 2 months, with 4 first-line antituberculous drugs having high CSF penetration (ussualy isoniazid, rifampicin, pyrazinamide, ethambutol) administered daily; the initial phase is followed by a *second phase* of another 10 months with only 2 first-line antituberculous drugs (isoniazid, rifampicin) administered 3 times per week [121]

2. *Controlled treatment* should approach:

- treatment adherence

- drug interactions and toxicities taking into consideration the followings (see table 3):a) the side effects to the antituberculous treatment are three times more frequent in HIV than non HIV patients; b) the interactions between the antituberculous and antiretroviral therapy may impede the administration of the most efficient regimen or a simultaneous therapy; the most important interaction involves the protease inhibitors (important class of antiretrovirals) and rifampicin (first line antituberculous drug). Rifampicin accelerates the hepatic metabolism of protease inhibitors decreasing their blood levels and increasing the risk of HIVdrug resistance. In addition protease inhibitors delay the metabolism of rifampicin increasing its serum concentration and toxicity. Izoniazid and rifampicin also decrease the concentration of fluconazole, an antifungal frequently used in the HIV patients. Additionally there are many other interactions between rifampicin and antiretrovirals, corticosteroids or trimetoprim/sulfamethoxazole (table 3). For this reason rifabutin is preferred to rifampicin in HIV patients along with a prolonged treatment.

- neurological/extraneurological complications

Monitoring for ensuing complications includes a complete physical examination, laboratory data, CSF aspects and imaging studies. It is important to consider the followings: a) neurological complications are more frequent in HIV patients (mostly due to immune exacerbation as tuberculous vasculopathy or IRIS); b) neurological complications may occur during treatment: hydrocephalus and arachnoiditis could sometimes occur even in the presence of a correct treatment; c) complications are frequently associated with other undetected TB localizations.

- drug resistance.

The risk of resistance is increased in non-adherent patients, large bacillary load and patients who start less efficient regimens. The glucocorticoid therapy reestablishes the low permeability of the blood-brain barrier and could therefore decrease the CSF diffusion of antibiotics. Inadequate doses of antituberculous therapy or low CSF antituberculous concentration may induce drug resistance. An unfavourable clinical evolution and decreasing CD4+T cell count require repeated CSF collection for culture and drug resistance. Close surveillance for drug resistance is essential throughout the entire course of therapy.

3. *Individualized treatment.* The patient's co-morbidities (like viral hepatitis or other risk factors for hepatotoxicity, ocular diseases, renal failure, allergic reactions,other medications and pregnancy) must be investigated before establishing the drug regimen and should continue to be closely monitored.

Treatment of tuberculomas. Cerebral tuberculomas are potentially curable tumor-like masses. There is a low number of tuberculoma cases reported in HIV patients [94- 95, 122-125]. Treatment is based on the same principles as TBM but with the following mentions:

- The perilesional granulomatous vasculitis decreases the penetration of antituberculous drugs; the lesions heal progressively and require 12 to 30 months of antituberculous treatment, or even longer;

- The recommended regimen is based on rifampicin, izoniazid and pirazinamide for 4 to 5 months and then rifampicin and izoniazid for 12 to 16 additional months. Other active drugs include rifabutin, fluoroquinolones, kanamycin, ethionamide;

- Surgical treatment is rarely needed; it is indicated in tuberculomas with mass effect, increased intracranial hypertension and hydrocephalus. The antituberculous treatment should be started before surgery. The recurrence after surgical ablation is unsual.

- Glucocorticoid therapy is an important part of the treatment regimen as it reduces the edema and improves the clinical manifestations. It should be maintained for at least 4 to 8 weeks.

Treatment monitoring requires the clinical and radiological follow-up on the long term. The evolution of other tuberculous localizations if present should also remain under observation. Response to therapy is favorable despite large lesions or immunodeficiency.

Treatment of tuberculous abscesses requires surgical and pharmacological treatment similar to the regimen recommended in tuberculoma but for an interval of 18 months to 2 years. The *prognosis* is unfavourable due to severe imunodeficiency and large lesions [99, 101].

Treatment of NTB with resistant strains of M.tbc. The risk of resistance is higher in geographic areas with high prevalence of resistant mycobacteria and in the case of recent TB improperly treated. Resistance could occur against one or more antituberculous drugs. The association between HIV and multidrug resistance (MDR-TB) or extensive drug resistance (XDR-TB) is not well documented [126,127].The antituberculous treatment should be undertaken according to the advice of an experienced specialist only and should include at least 4 antituberculous drugs with an increased diffusion in the CSF [128].

Treatment of CNS TB with nontuberculous myobacteria. Data related to infections with nontuberculous mycobacteria is scarce and insufficient for establishing definite treatment guidelines. Therefore treatment regimens are largely undefined and the subsequent outcome remains disappointing. The severity of the evolution appears to be related to the variable sensitivity to the antituberculous antibiotics and the advanced stages of immunodeficiency which predispose to a disseminated disease. Therapeutic regimens should be individualized to include complex drug associations (5-6 drugs) on longer periods of time. A close consultation with an experienced specialist is required. Mycobacteria belonging to the MAC display increased resistance against most antituberculous drugs and therefore a large variety of therapeutic regimens was evaluated. The repeated therapeutic failure is apparently linked to the diverse sensitivity to antituberculous drugs associated with M. avium species. Moreover there is the alternative that some HIV patients could be simultaneously infected with more than one species of M avium. Macrolides proved efficient but cannot penetrate to the CSF. Chlaritromycin is involved in several drug interactions with the antiretroviral therapy. Considering the increased risk for disseminated forms induced by the MAC it is recommended to add azithromycin, ethambutol and rifabutin to therapy. Other drugs that could be associated in such cases include fluoroquinolones, streptomycin, amikacin. Treatment should always be based on the results of susceptibility testing. After 12 months of treatment, prophylaxis with macrolides is recommended until the CD4+ count raises above 100/mm3.M. scrofulaceum, M. simiae, M. malmoense reveal the same sensitivity pattern as MAC. In the case of M. kansasii recommended drugs include: rifabutin, streptomycin, HIN, ethambutol, amikacin.

Treatment during Pregnancy. The antituberculous treatment is urgently instituted according to classic treatment regimens. Among prohibited drugs are streptomycin, fluoroquinolones and ethionamide.

Treatment of NeuroIRIS-TB. Neurologic TB-IRIS is a rare manifestation of TB-IRIS. It generally occurs within 2-3 months after initiating the combination of antiretroviral and the antituberculous therapy [42].The risk of IRIS increases with the early starting and high efficacy of antiretroviral therapy. Delaying the antiretroviral therapy with a minimum of 2 weeks after antituberculous therapy is recommended to avoid IRIS complication. Usually IRIS is self-limited and requires symptomatic or anti-inflammatory treatment without stopping the antiretroviral treatment. Severe forms benefit from treatment with prednisone or methylpred-nisolone 1 mg/g gradually tapered within the 2 following weeks [129,130]

8.2. The antiretroviral therapy

The antiretroviral (ARV) treatment ought to be started as soon as possible after the antituberculous treatment. The urgency of the ARV therapy increases with the degree of immunodeficiency. Three important studies (CAMELIA performed in Cambodgia, SAPiT conducted in South Africa and STRIDE a multinational study) established that an earlier start of the ARV therapy significantly decreases the mortality in AIDS patients and especially in patients in which the CD4+ cell count is below <50 cells /mm³. Although the development of IRIS is more frequent if the ARV treatment is more precocious, the gravity of the IRIS manifestations in the 3 studies above cannot justify a longer delay of the antiretroviral therapy. Most guidelines recommended that HIV patients start the antiretroviral treatment at least 2 weeks after the antituberculous treatment if the CD4+ count is below 50 cells per mm³ ; the antiretroviral treatment can be delayed until 4 weeks if the CD4+ count > 50 cells/mm³. Note that NTB in HIV patients could be shadowed by the possible reactivation of other neurotropic agents (cytomegalovirus, toxoplasma, JV virus) or cerebral tumors (cerebral lymphoma, Kaposi sarcoma).The diagnosis in these cases could be difficult and if these associations are not excluded from diagnosis, treatment should also address these conditions with the risk of multiple drug interactions. Such is the case of cerebral toxoplasmosis.

- **The main characteristics of antiretroviral treatment in HIV patients with NTB**

  o Therapeutic regimens must contain antiretroviral drugs with a high penetration in the CSF. The main ARV drugs used in the co-infection with TB are listed in table 3 along with their adverse reacions.

  o The antiretroviral therapy in NTB is based on reverse transcriptase inhibitors represented by 2 important classes: nucleoside reverse transcriptase inhibitors (NRTI) and non-nucleoside reverse transcriptase inhibitors (NNRTI). The highest drug penetration into the CSF is assigned to zidovudine, abacavir, nevirapine, delavirdine. Although efavirenz (a NNRTI) does not display high levels in the CSF some studies advocate a very good response in the treated adults [131]. Protease inhibitors should not be used due to their interaction with rifampicin and low diffusion in the CSF. If their use is required (as a result of resistance or toxicity to other antiretrovirals) rifampicin is to be replaced with rifabutin with similar results.

  o The doses of antiretrovirals should be changed according to the antituberculous drug interference.

- **Factors to consider**

1. *Combined treatment* includes 3 NNRTIs with a preferred option for trizivir (combination of zidovudine, abacavir and lamivudine) or 2 NRTIs + 1 NNRTI (ussualy efavirenz).

2. *Controlled treatment* should approach:

- The adherence (especially if a large number of drugs are introduced at the same time) [132]. Nevertheless adherence to trizivir is high (the number of capsules is low, there are few adverse reactions).

- Drug interactions and toxicities (see table 3). The clinician should recognize the overlapping toxicities, drug interactions and also the occurrence of IRIS (paradoxical reactions) [133].The interactions between NNRTI or NRTI and antituberculous drugs are few. The risk of toxicity is minimal but adverse reactions are possible with some NRTIs (see table 3). Regarding the toxicity the ARV could interfere not only with antituberculous drugs but also with other drugs used in the prophylaxis or treatment of other opportunistic infections (such as fluconazol for Candida or Criptococcus neoformans or sulphametoxazole/trimethoprim for Penumocystis jirovecii).

- The efficiency and complications of treatment. The efficiency is to be monitored on a clinical, virologic and immunological basis. The best control in HIV infections is the virologic (RNA HIV viral load) and immunologic control (CD4+ cell count).Treatment control could be undertaken at 14 days, one month, three and six months respectively. If the HIV RNA load does not become undetectable after 3 months of treatment virologic failure should be considered. If this is the case investigations on the underlying cause should focus on the lack of adherence, acquired resistance (especially to NNRTIs) or a wrong treatment regimen (doses, antagonistic associations or the lack of drug penetration to the CSF). Nevertheless the intracerebral load of HIV could be hard to evaluate since the viral load detection in the serum does not always reflect the intracerebral levels of HIV.

- Drug resistance. In case of virologic failure drug-resistance testing should be obtained during treatment with the failing ARV regimen or within 4 weeks of treatment discontinuation. Resistance to antiretrovirals generally applies to most compounds in the same class.A new regimen with other fully active drugs preferably from other new classes must be restarted.

3. *Individualized treatment*: the treatment options should address other opportunistic infections and the patient's medical history. A CD4+ count under 200 cells/mm³ urges the prophylaxis against fungal infections (cryptococcus, pneumocytsis). Prophylaxis against toxoplasmosis should be started at a CD4+ cell count under 100 cells/mm³ due to an increased risk of reactivation. Pregnant patients require urgent ARV treatment after 14 days of antituberculous treatment.

9. Conclusion

The failure of the antituberculous/antiretroviral treatment is generally a result of the low compliance, inadequate treatment regimen (length, doses, low penetration into the CSF, adverse reactions impeding the use of certain efficacious drugs), delays in the diagnosis or treatment resistance. Any changes in the clinical examination, imaging studies and CSF aspect during treatment or at follow-up require further investigations. Despite the immunodeficiency the prognosis of CNS TB in HIV patients resembles that of non-HIV patients.

ANTITUBERCULOUS DRUGS		
Drug	Pharmacologic aspects	Drug interactions/Adverse reactions
Isoniazid (NIH)*** (first-line agent)	Interferes with mycolic acids synthesis. Bactericidal to rapidly-dividing extracellular mycobacteria, bacteriostatic against the slow-growing intracellular mycobacteria. CSF peak concentrations exceed 30 times the minimal inhibitory concentration	Peripheral neuropathy (requires pyridoxine supplementation). Hepatotoxicity (reversible) depending on the dose and association with rifampicin and alcohol consumption. Rare cases of fulminant hepatitis. Rare allergic reactions.
Rifampicin* (first-line agent) Associations of rifampicin: rifamate, rifater Rifabutin* Rifapentine is a semi-synthetic rifamycin derivate with longer half-time (not recommended in HIV patients)	Rifampicin acts against intra and extracellular bacilli, especially on slow-growing mycobacteria (bactericidal). The metabolism is primarily hepatic; because of its ability to induce certain microsomal hepatic enzymes (CYP3A4) it interferes with the metabolism of other drugs. Poorly penetrates the CSF in the absence of meningeal inflammation. In meningitis CSF level is up to 10-20% of the serum levels. Rapid emergence of resistant mycobacteria. Rifabutin is bactericidal.The level of rifabutin in the serum is 7-10 times lower than the concentration of rifampicin. It easily diffuses through the uninflammed meninges.	Renal failure. Digestive and allergic reactions. Hepatotoxicity (cholestatic hepatitis) especially in drug associations. Hemorrhagic manifestations due to thrombocytopenia. Sulfamethoxazole/ trimethoprim enhances the effect of rifampicin and could increase its toxicity. Corticosteroids decrease the level of rifampicin. Rifampicin could singnificantly reduce the plasma concentrations of most PIs and some NNRTIs; it could be associated with NRTI and some NNRTIs. Adverse reactions to rifabutin mirror those of rifampicin; in addition rifabutin could induce uveitis, arthralgias, leucopenia, asymptomatic hepatitis. Rifabutin does not interact with PIs. Because rifabutin is a less potent inducer, it is generally considered a reasonable alternative to rifampicin. Doses should be adjusted in the coadministration with an PI ; underdosing of rifabutin can result in selection of rifamycin resistance, whereas overdosing of rifabutin might result in toxicities.
Pyrazinamide*** (first-line agent)	Active against intracellular bacilli only at acid pH. Bactericidal/bacteriostatic (dose dependent). Is well absorbed and crosses the blood-brain barrier leading to CSF concentrations almost as high as those in the blood	Hepatotoxicity Hypersensitivity reactions
Ethambutol* (first-line agent)	Bactericidal with low activity. Ethambutol could increase the activity of other antituberculous drugs affecting the cellular permeability of MAC strains and possibly of multiresistant M.tbc strain. Low CSF level (moderate rise above the minimum bactericidal concentration)	Optic neuropathy especially after prolonged treatments. Rarely triggers allergic reactions and hyperuricemia. No hepatotoxicity reactions.
Streptomycin* (second-line drug)	Belongs to aminoglycosides class. Bactericidal. Active only on replicating extracellular bacilli. Poor CSF level even in patients with meningitis. High rate of resistance	Nephrotoxicity. Neurotoxicity. Ototoxicity. Contraindicated in pregnancy. No recorded hepatotoxic reactions
Amikacin* (second-line drug)	Belongs to the class of aminoglycosides. The same characteristics as streptomycin. Low CSF concentrations	Less toxic than streptomycin.Contraindicated in pregnancy

ANTITUBERCULOUS DRUGS		
Drug	Pharmacologic aspects	Drug interactions/Adverse reactions
Ofloxacin** Levofloxacin** Moxifloxacin** Ciprofloxacin *	Belongs to fluorochinolones class. Bactericidal. Active on rapidly multiplying bacilli. Acts on nontuberculous mycobacteria. Good CSF penetrations. except for ciprofloxacin	Rare adverse reactions. To be avoided in pregnancy. Interferes with antiacids
Azithromycin Clarithromycin	Belongs to macrolides class. Bacteriostatic. Active on nontuberculous mycobacteria. High intracellular levels Do not cross the blood brain barrier.	Clarithromycin interfers with PIs and efavirenz; azithromycin does not display these interferences.
Ethionamide*** (second-line drug)	Bacteriostatic/bactericidal (dose depending). Effect on extra/intra cellular bacilli. Good CSF penetration (equal to those in serum).Active on resistant mycobacteria.	Allergic reactions. Digestive reactions. Hepatotoxicity. Neurotoxicity. Teratogenic effects
Cycloserine*** (second-line drug)	Bactericidal/bacteriostatic (dose depending). Effect on intra and extracellular bacilli, including resistant mycobacteria. Good CSF penetration	Neuropsy-chic reactions. Rash. Not recommended with efavirenz. No hepatotoxicity; indicated in patients with acute hepatitis in combination with other nonhepatotoxic drugs.
CCR5 antagonist: maraviroc (MVC) **	Belongs to the entry inhibitor class (chemokine receptor antagonist); it blocks HIV entry into the host cell. Substrate of CYP3A enzymes.	Hepatotoxicity. Rash. Caution and dose adjustment is necessary when MVC is used in combination with CYP3A inducers agents (such as EFV or rifampin).
Fusion inhibitor: enfuvirtide (EFV) *	Belongs to the entry inhibitor class. It is not affected by the CYP enzymes	Hypersensitivity reactions. Can be used with the rifamycins
Integrase inhibitor: RAL**	HIV-1 integrase inhibitor. Blood-brain-barrier restrict RAL entry; meningeal inflammation enhances drug entry.	Hypersensitivity reactions. Rifampin and rifabutin can significantly reduce the concentration of RAL.
Protease inhibitors (PI): SQV*;ATV***;DRV*;FPV***; AMP ***; IDV***; LPV***; NFV*;RTV*; TPV*	Interfere with the protease enzyme that HIV uses to produce infectious viral particles. PI are CYP P450 inducer and substrate	Hepatotoxicity (requires monitoring of hepatic enzymes). Rash. Prolonged QT interval. PIs are not recommended with rifampicin. Adjust the dose of PIs when combined with rifabutin
Non-nucleoside reverse transcriptase inhibitors (NNRTI): EFV**;NVP*** ETV; DVR***	NNRTI bind to revers transcriptase, interfering with its ability to convert the HIV RNA into HIV DNA The NNRTIs are also substrates of CYP3A4 and can act as an inducer/inhibitor or mixt NNRTIs are related with an increased risk of resistance if the therapeutic regimen is not respected.	Hepatotoxicity. Hypersensitivity reactions. Fewer interactions with RIF; nevirapine does not affect the levels of RIF; efavirenz or nevirapine-based regimen are preffered when using associated therapy with RIF; etravirine not recommended with RIF. Adjust the doses in the combination of EFV and rifabutin /rifampicine
Nucleos(t)ide reverse transcriptase inhibitors (NRTI): ZDV***; 3TC** ABC ***; d4T ** ddI* ; FTC**TDF*; ZAL*	Interfere with reverse transcription and conversion of HIV RNA to HIV-DNA. Do not use the CYP metabolic pathway. No significant interaction with rifampicin or rifabutin	Hepatitis. Neuropathy (only stavudine, didanosine). Optic neuritis (didanosine)

***very good ability to cross the blood-brain barrier; ** moderate ability to cross the blood-brain barrier; * low ability to cross the blood-brain barrier

Table 3. The most important antituberculous and antiretroviral drugs used in the treatment of CNS tuberculosis [113-118]

Acknowledgements

The authors wish to express special thanks to professor Ionescu Virgil for the MRI reproductions and their interpretation.

Author details

Simona Alexandra Iacob[1] and Diana Gabriela Iacob[2]

1 National Institute of Infectious Diseases "Matei Bals" Bucharest, Romania

2 "Carol Davila" University of Medicine and Pharmacie, Bucharest, Romania

References

[1] Merrill S, Introduction to Syndemics: A Systems Approach to Public and Community Health. San Francisco, CA: Jossey-Bass. 2009

[2] Farer L.S, Lowell A.M, Meador M.P. Extrapulmonary TB in the United States. Am. J. Epidemiol. 1979;109:205-217

[3] A Kenyan British Medical Research Council Co-opertive Investigation. TB in Kenya 1984: a third national survey and a comparison with earlier surveys in 1964 and 1974. Tubercle. 1989; 70: 5-20

[4] Thwaites G, Fisher M, Hemingway C, Scott G, Solomon T, et al. British Infection Society guidelines for the diagnosis and treatment of TB of the central nervous system in adults and children. J Infect 2009; 59: 167–187

[5] Berenguer J, Moreno S, Laguna F, et al. Tuberculous meningitis in patients infected with the human immunodeficiency virus. N Engl J Med 1992; 326:668-672.

[6] Shafer R.W, Edlin B.R.TB in patients infected with human immunodeficiency virus: perspective on the past decade. Clin. Infect. Dis. 1996; 22:683-704.

[7] Whiteman M, Espinoza L, Post M.J, Bell M.D, Falcone S. Central nervous system TB in HIV-infected patients: Clinical and radiographic findings. AJNR Am J Neuroradiol 1995;16:1319-1327.

[8] Katrak S.M, Shembalkar P.K, Bijwe S.R, Bhandarkar L.D.The clinical, radiological and pathological profile of tuberculous meningitis in patients with and without human immunodeficiency virus infection. J Neurol Sci. 2000 Dec 1;181(1-2):118-126.

[9]   Shaw J.E.T,Pasipanodya J.G, Gumba T. Meningeal TB: High Long-Term Mortality Despite Standard Therapy Medicine: 2010; 89(3): 189-195

[10] Rock R.B, Olin M, Baker C.A, Molitor T.W, Peterson P.K. Central nervous system TB: Pathogenesis and clinical aspects. Clin Microbiol Rev 2008;21:243-261.

[11] Garg R.K. TB of the central nervous system, Postgrad Med J. 1999;75:133-140.

[12] Donald P.R, Schoeman JF. Tuberculous meningitis. N Engl J Med. 2004;351:1719-1720.

[13] Sanduzzi A, Fraziano M, Mariani F.Monocytes/macrophages in HIV infection and TB. J Biol Regul Homeost Agents. 2001 Jul-Sep;15(3):294-298.

[14] Barnes P.F, Bloch A.B, Davidson P.T, Snider D. E.TB in patients with human immunodeficiency virus infection. N Engl J Med. 1991;324:1644–1650.

[15] Flynn J.L, Goldstein M.M, Chan J, Triebold K.J, Pfeffer K, Lowenstein C.J, Schreiber R, Mak T.W, Bloom B.R. Tumor necrosis factor-alpha is required in the protective immune response against Mycobacterium TB in mice. Immunity. 1995 Jun;2(6):561-572

[16] Flynn J.L, Chan J,Triebold K.J,Dalton D.K,Stewart T.A, B R Bloom B.R. An essential role for interferon-γ in resistance to Mycobacterium TB infection J. Exp. Med. 1995; 178:2249–2254.

[17] Fenton, M.J, Vermeulen MW, Kim, Burdick SM, Strieter R.M, Kornfeld H. Induction of gamma interferon production in human alveolar macrophages by Mycobacterium TB. Infect. Immun.1999; 65:5149– 5156.

[18] Keane J, Gershon S, Wise RP, Mirabile-Levens E, John Kasznica J, et al. TB associated with infliximab, a tumor necrosis factor α-neutralizing agent. N Engl J Med. 2001;345(15):1098–1104.

[19] Caruso A.M, Serbina N, Klein E, Triebold K, Bloom B.R, Flynn J.L. Mice deficient in CD4 T cells have only transiently diminished levels of IFN-γ, yet succumb to TB. J. Immunol. 1999;162:5407–5416.

[20] Adams L.B, Mason C.M, Kolls J.K, Scollard D, Krahenbuhl J.L, Nelson S.Exacerbation of acute and chronic murine TB by administration of a tumor necrosis factor receptor-expressing adenovirus. J. Infect. Dis. 1995; 171:400–405.

[21] Cooper A.M, Dalton D.K, Stewart T.A, Griffin J.P, Russell D.G, Orme I.M. Disseminated TB in IFN-γ gene-disrupted mice J. Exp. Med. 1993;178:2243–2248.

[22] Silver R.F, Li Q, Ellner J.J. Expression of virulence of Mycobacterium TB within human monocytes: virulence correlates with intracellular growth and induction of tumor necrosis factor alpha but not with evasion of lymphocyte-dependent monocyte effector functions. Infect Immun. 1998;66(3):1190-1199.

[23] Brian R, Lane B.R, Markovitz D,M, Woodford N,L, Rochford R, Strieter R, Coffey M. TNF-α Inhibits HIV-1 Replication in Peripheral Blood Monocytes and Alveolar Mac-

rophages by Inducing the Production of RANTES and Decreasing C-C Chemokine Receptor 5 (CCR5) Expression.The Journal of Immunology 1999; 163 (7): 3653-3661.

[24] Osborn L, Kunkel S, Nabel G.Tumor necrosis factor α and interleukin 1 stimulate human immunodeficiency virus enhancer by activation of the nuclear factor κB. Proc. Natl. Acad. Sci. USA. 1989;86: 2336-2340.

[25] Wallis R.S, Wjeka M, Amir-Tahmasseb M. Influence of TB on human immunodeficiency virusenhanced citokineexpressionand elevated b2 microglobulinin HIV associated tubercuosis, J Inf. Dis, 1993;167:43-48.

[26] Nagesh Babu G, Kumar A, Kalita J, Misra UK.,Proinflammatory cytokine levels in the serum and cerebrospinal fluid of tuberculous meningitis patients. Neurosci Lett. 2008;436(1):48-51.

[27] Mastroiani C.M, Paoletii F, Lichtner M, Dágostino C, Vullo V, Delia S. Cerebrospinal fluid cytokines in patients with tuberculous meningitis.Clin Immunol.immunopathol.1997;84(2):171-6

[28] Tsenova L, Bergtold A, Freedman V.H, Young R.A, Kaplan G. Tumor necrosis factor alpha is a determinant of pathogenesis and disease progression in mycobacterial infection in the central nervous system. Proc Natl Acad Sci U S A. 1999; 96(10): 5657-5662.

[29] Schoeman J.F, Ravenscroft A, Hartzenberg H.B. Possible role of adjunctive thalidomide therapy in the resolution of a massive intracranial tuberculous abscess. Childs Nerv Syst. 2001;17(6):370-372.

[30] Schoeman J.F, Fieggen G, Seller N, Mendelson M, Hartzenberg B. Intractable intracranial tuberculous infection responsive to thalidomide: report of four cases. J Child Neurol. 2006 Apr;21(4):301-308

[31] Schoeman J.F, Andronikou S, Stefan D.C, Freeman N, van Toorn R. Tuberculous meningitis-related optic neuritis: recovery of vision with thalidomide in 4 consecutive cases. J Child Neurol. 2010;25(7):822-828.

[32] Sinha M.K, Garg R.K, Anuradha H.K, Agarwal A, Parihar A, Mandhani P.A,Paradoxical vision loss associated with optochiasmatic tuberculoma in tuberculous, J Child Neurol. 2010;25(7):822-828.

[33] Jacobs M, Togbe D, Fremond C, Samarina A, Allie N, Botha T. M. Tumor necrosis factor is critical to control TB infection. Microbes Infect. 2007 Apr;9(5):623-628.

[34] Patel V.B,Bhigjee A.l, Bill P.L.A,Connolly C.A.Cytokine profiles in HIV seropositive patients with tuberculous meningitis,J Neurol Neurosurg Psychiatry 2002;73:5 598-599

[35] Fischer, H.-G, Reichmann G.Brain dendritic cells and macrophages/microglia in central nervous system inflammation. J. Immunol. 2001;166:2717-2726.

[36] Cosenza M.A, Zhao M.L, Si Q, Lee S.C.. Human brain parenchymal Mricroglia express CD14 and CD45 and are productively infected by HIV-1 in HIV-1 encephalitis. Brain Pathol. 200;12:442-455

[37] Curto M, Reali C, Palmieri G, Scintu F, Schivo ML, Sogos V. Marcialis MA, Ennas M.G, Schwarz H, Pozzi G, Gremo F.Inhibition of cytokines expression in human microglia infected by virulent and non-virulent mycobacteria. Neurochem. Int. 2004;44:381-392.

[38] Lee J, Ling C, Michelle M, Kosmalski M, Hulseberg P, Schreiber H.A. Intracerebral Mycobacterium bovis bacilli Calmette-Guerin infection-induced immune responses in the CNS. J Neuroimmunol. 2009 ;18;213(1-2):112-122

[39] Rock R.B, Hu S, Gekker G, Sheng W.S, May B, Phillip K. V.P,Kapur P, Mycobacterium TB–Induced Cytokine and Chemokine Expression by Human Microglia and Astrocytes: Effects of Dexamethasone J Infect Dis. 2005; 192 (12): 2054-2058.

[40] Peterson P.K, Gekker G, Hu S, Sheng W.S, Anderson W.R. CD14 receptor-mediated uptake of nonopsonized Mycobacterium TB by human microglia. Infect Immun. 1995;63(4):1598-1602.

[41] Be N.A, Kim K.S, Bishai W.R, Jain S.K. Pathogenesis of central nervous system TB. Curr Mol Med. 2009;9:94–99.

[42] Pepper D.J, Marais S, Maartens G, Rebe K, Morroni C, Rangaka M.X, Oni T, Wilkinson R.J, Meintjes G. Neurologic manifestations of paradoxical TB associated immune reconstitution inflammatory syndrome:a case series. Clin Infect Dis. 2009;48:e96–107.

[43] World Health Organization.Antiretroviral therapy for HIV infection in adults and adolescents: recommendations for a public health approach: 2010 revision. Geneva, Switzerland: World Health Organization; 2010.

[44] Bourgarit A, Carcelain G, Martinez V, Lascoux C, Delcey V, Gicquel B, Vicaut E, Lagrange P.H, Sereni D, Autran B. Explosion of tuberculin-specific Th1-responses induces immune restoration syndrome in TB and HIV co-infected patients. AIDS. 2006; ; 9;20(2):F1-7.

[45] Tan D.B, Yong Y.K, Tan H.Y, Kamarulzaman A, Tan L.H, Lim A, James I, French M, Price P. HIV Med. Immunological profiles of immune restoration disease presenting as mycobacterial lymphadenitis and cryptococcal meningitis 2008 ;9(5):307-316.

[46] Oliver B.G, Elliott J.H, Price P, Phillips M, Cooper D.A, French M.A, TB after commencing antiretroviral therapy for HIV infection is associated with elevated CXCL9 and CXCL10 responses to Mycobacterium TB antigens.J Acquir Immune Defic Syndr. 2012; Jun Epub ahead of print

[47] Algood H.M.S, Chan J, Flynn J.L Chemokines and TB.Cytokine & Growth Factor Rev 2003; 14: 467-477.

[48] Kremlev S.G, Roberts R.L, Palmer C. Differential expression of chemokines and chemokine receptors during microglial activation and inhibition. J Neuroimmunol. 2004;149(1-2):1-9.

[49] Simonney N, Dewulf G, Herrmann J.L, Gutierrez M.C, Vicaut E.Anti-PGL-Tb1 responses as an indicator of the immune restoration syndrome in HIV-TB patients. TB (Edinb).2008;88: 453–461.

[50] Cheng V.C.C, Yuen K, Chan W.M, Vong.SS, Ma E.S.K, Khan R.M.T. Immune disease involving the innate and adaptive response. Clin Infect Dis. 2000;30:882-892.

[51] Foudraine N.A, Hovenkamp E, Notermans D.W, Immunopathology as a result of highly active antiretroviral therapy in HIV-infected patients. AIDS. 1999;13:177-184.

[52] Wilkinson K.A, Meintjes G, Seldon R, Goliath R, Wilkinson R.J. Immunological characterisation of an unmasking TB-IRIS case. S Afr Med J. 2012; 2;102(6):512-517.

[53] Price- Elliott J.H, Vohith K, Saramony S, Savuth C, Dara C, Sarim C, Huffam S.Immunopathogenesis and diagnosis of TB and TB-associated immune reconstitution inflammatory syndrome during early antiretroviral therapy. J Infect Dis. 2009; 200(11): 1736-1745

[54] Haddow L.J, Dibben O, Moosa M.Y, Borrow P, Easterbrook P.J.Circulating inflammatory biomarkers can predict and characterize TB-associated immune reconstitution inflammatory syndrome. AIDS. 2011; 25(9):1163-1174.

[55] Conradie F, Foulkes A.S, Ive P, Yin X, Roussos K, Glencross D.K, Lawrie D. Natural killer cell activation distinguishes Mycobacterium TB-mediated immune reconstitution syndrome from chronic HIV and HIV/MTB co-infection. J Acquir Immune Defic Syndr. 2011;58(3):309-318

[56] Caws M, Thwaites G, Stepniewska K, Nguyen Thi Ngoc Lan, Nguyen Thi Hong Duyen. Beijing Genotype of Mycobacterium TB Is Significantly Associated with Human Immunodeficiency Virus Infection and Multidrug Resistance in Cases of Tuberculous. J Clin Microbiol. 2006 ; 44(11): 3934–3939

[57] Horsburgh C.R.. Mycobacterium avium complex infection in the acquired immunodeficiency syndrome. N Engl J Med. 1991;324:1332-1338

[58] Yakrus M.A, Reeves M.W, Hunter S.B. Characterization of isolates of Mycobacterium avium serotypes 4 and 8 from patients with AIDS by multilocus enzyme electrophoresis. J. Clin. Microbiol. 1992; 30:6 1474-1478

[59] Zeller V, Nardi A.L, Truffot-Pernot C, Sougakoff W, Stankoff B. Katlama C, Bricaire F. Disseminated Infection with a Mycobacterium Related to Mycobacterium triplex with Central Nervous System Involvement Associated with AIDS Clin. Microbiol. 2003; vol. 41 (6):2785-2787

[60] Bermudez LE. Eur J Clin Microbiol Infect Dis. Immunobiology of Mycobacterium avium infection. 1994; 13(11):1000-1006.

[61] Kallenius G, T. Koivula K. J. Rydgard S.E. Hoffner A. Valentin B. Asjoe C. Ljungh, U. Sharma, Svenson SB. Human immunodeficiency virus type 1 enhances intracellular growth of Mycobacterium avium in human macrophages. Infect. Immun.1992; 60:2453-2458.

[62] Hartmann P, Plum G.Immunological defense mechanisms in TB and MAC infection, Diagn.Microbiol.Infect.Dis, 1999;34,147-15.

[63] Flor A, Capdevila J.A, Martin N, Gavalda J, Pahissa A. Nontuberculous Mycobacterial Meningitis: Report of Two Cases and Review, Clinical Infectious Diseases 1996; 23:1266-1273.

[64] Jacob C.N, Henein S.S, Heurich D.E, Kamholz S. Nontuberculous mycobacterial infection of the central nervous system in patients with AIDS. South Med J. 1993;86:638-640.

[65] Jacob C., S. Henein A. Heurich, Kamholz S. 1991. Nontuberculous mycobacterial meningitis in patients with AIDS. Am. Rev. Respir. Dis.; 143:279A.

[66] Uldry PA, J. Bogousslavsky F, Regli J.P, Chave, Beer V.Chronic Mycobacterium-avium complex infection of the central nervous system in a nonimmunosuppressed woman Eur. Neurol. 1992;32:285-288.

[67] Karstaedt A.S, Valtchanova S, Barriere R, Crewe-Brown HR.Tuberculous meningitis in South African urban adults. QJM 1998;91:743-747.

[68] Thwaites G.E, Duc Bang N, Huy Dung N, Thi Quy H, Thi Tuong Oanh D. The influence of HIV infection on clinical presentation, response to treatment, and outcome in adults with Tuberculous meningitis. J Infect Dis. 2005; 15;192(12):2134-2141.

[69] Karande S, Gupta V, Kulkarni M, Joshi A, Rele M.Tuberculous meningitis and HIV. Indian J Pediatr. 2005;72(9):755-760

[70] Schutte C.M. Clinical, cerebrospinal fluid and pathological findings and outcomes in HIV-positive and HIV-negative patients with tuberculous meningitis.Infection. 2001;29(4):213-217.

[71] Bergemann A, Karstaedt AS. The spectrum of meningitis in a population with high prevalence of HIV disease. Q J Med. 1996;89:499–504.

[72] Rana F.S, Hawken M.P, Mwachari C, Bhatt S.M, Abdullah F. Autopsy study of HIV-1-positive and HIV-1-negative adult medical patients in Nairobi, Kenya. J Acquir Immune Defic Syndr. 2000;24(1):23-29.

[73] Maniar J.K., Kamath R.R., Mandalia S.Shah K,Maniar A.HIV and TB: partners in crime Indian J Dermatol Venereol Leprol. 2006; 72:276-282.

[74] Ige O.M, Sogaolu O.M, Ogunlade O.A. Pattern of presentation of TB and the hospital prevalence of TB and HIV co-infection in University College Hospital, Ibadan: a review of five years (1998 - 2002). Afr J Med Med Sci. 2005; 34:329-333.

[75] Laguna F, Adrados M, Ortega A, Gonzalez-Lahoz JM.Tuberculous meningitis with acellular cerebrospinal fluid in AIDS patients.AIDS, 1992:6;1165-1167.

[76] Guy E. Thwaites The Influence of HIV Infection on Clinical Presentation, Response to Treatment, and Outcome in Adults with TBM *J Infect Dis.* (2005) 192 (12): 2134-2141)

[77] El Sahly H.M, Teeter L.D, Pan X, Musser J.M, Graviss EA.Mortality associated with central nervous system TB. J Infect. 2007;55: 502–509.

[78] Bernaerts A, Vanhoenacker F.M, Parizel P.M, Van Goethem J.W, Van Altena R, Laridon A, De Roeck J, Coeman V, De Schepper AM. TB of the central nervous system: overview of neuroradiological findings. Eur Radiol. 2003 Aug;13(8):1876-1890.

[79] Kumar R, Kohli N, Thavnani H, Kumar A, Sharma B. Value of CT scan in the diagnosis of meningitis. Indian Pediatr. 1996;33(6):465-468.

[80] Verdon R, Chevret S, Laissy JP, Wolff M.Tuberculous meningitis in adults: review of 48 cases. Clin Infect Dis. 1996;22(6):982-8

[81] Dubé M.P, Holtom P.D, Larsen R.A.Tuberculous meningitis in patients with and without human immunodeficiency virus infection. Am J Med. 1992;93(5):520-524.

[82] Torok M.E, Kambugu A, Wright E.Immune reconstitution disease of the central nervous system. Curr Opin HIV AIDS. 2008; 3(4):438-445.

[83] Narotam P.K, Kemp M, Buck R, Gouws E, van Dellen J.R, Bhoola K.D. Hyponatremic natriuretic syndrome in tuberculous meningitis: the probable role of atrial natriuretic peptide. Neurosurgery. 1994;34:982-988.

[84] Tang W.W, Kaptein E.M, Feinstein EI, Massry S.G. Hyponatraemia in hospitalized patients with the acquired immunodeficiency syndrome (AIDS) and the AIDS-related complex. Am J Med. 1993;94:169-174.

[85] Puccioni-Sohler Marzia, Brandão Carlos Otávio. Factors associated to the positive cerebrospinal fuid culture in the tuberculous meningitis. Arq. Neuro-Psiquiatr. 2007; 65(1): 48-53.

[86] Thwaites G.E, Chau T.T, Farrar J.J. Improving the bacteriological diagnosis of tuberculous meningitis. J Clin Microbiol. 2004; 42(1):378-379.

[87] Tuon F.F, Higashino H.R, Lopes M.I, Litvoc M.N, Atomiya A.N, Antonangelo L, Leite O.M. Adenosine deaminase and tuberculous meningitis--a systematic review with meta-analysis. Scand J Infect Dis. 2010;42(3):198-207.

[88] Patel V.B, Singh R, Connoly C, Kasprowicz V,Thumbi N, Keertan D. Comparative Utility of Cytokine Levels and Quantitative RD-1-Specific T Cell Responses for Rapid

Immunodiagnosis of Tuberculous Meningitis. J Clin Microbiol. 2011 November; 49(11): 3971–3976.

[89] Flores L.L, Steingart KR, Dendukuri N, Schiller I, Minion J, Pai M, Ramsay A. HenryM. Systematic Review and Meta-Analysis of Antigen Detection Tests for the Diagnosis of TB. Clin Vaccine Immunol October 2011; 18 (10) 1616-1627.

[90] Scarpellini P, Racca S, Cinque P, Delfanti F, Gianotti N, Terreni MR, Vago L, Lazzarin A. Nested polymerase chain reaction for diagnosis and monitoring treatment response in AIDS patients with tuberculous meningitis. AIDS. 1995 ;9(8):895-900.

[91] Takahashi T, Tamura M, Takasu T.Tuberc Res Treat. The PCR-Based Diagnosis of Central Nervous System TB: Up to Date.2012; 2012:831292. Epub 2012 May 13.

[92] Thwaites GE, Chau TT, Caws M, Phu NH, Chuong LV.Isoniazid resistance, mycobacterial genotype and outcome in Vietnamese adults with tuberculous meningitis. Int J Tuberc Lung Dis 2002;6:865-71

[93] Thwaites GE, Nguyen DB, Nguyen HD, Hoang TQ, Do TT, Nguyen TC, Dexamethasone for the treatment of tuberculous meningitis in adolescents and adults. N Engl J Med. 2004 Oct 21;351(17):1741-51.

[94] Muin I.A, Zurin AR. Pulmonary miliary TB with multiple intracerebral tuberculous granulomas--report of two cases. Br J Neurosurg. 1998;12(6):585-587.

[95] Lecuit M, Rogeaux O, Bricaire F, Gentilini M.Intracerebral tuberculoma in HIV infection. Epidemiology and contribution of magnetic resonance imaging. Presse Med. 1994;23(19):891-895.

[96] Vidal J.E, Cimerman S, Silva P.R, Sztajnbok J, Coelho J.F, Lins D.L. Tuberculous brain abscess in a patient with AIDS: case report and literature review. Rev Inst Med Trop Sao Paulo. 2003;45:111-114

[97] Smith A.B, Smirniotopoulos J.G, Rushing E.J. From the archives of the AFIP: central nervous system infections associated with human immunodeficiency virus infection: radiologic-pathologic correlation. Radiographics. 2008;28(7):2033-2058.

[98] Farrar D.J, Timothy P, Flanigan, Gordon N.M, Gold R.L, Rich J.D. Tuberculous brain abscess in a patient with HIV infection: case report and review. Am J Med. 1997;102(3):297-301.

[99] Bottieau E, Noe A, Florence E, Colebunders R Multiple tuberculous brain abscesses in an HIV-infected patient successfully treated with HAART and antituberculous treatment. Infection. 2003; 31(2):118-120.

[100] Whiteman M.L. Neuroimaging of central nervous system TB in HIV-infected patients. Neuroimaging Clin N Am 1997;7:199-213.

[101] Kaushik K, Karade S, Kumar S, Kapila K. Tuberculous brain abscess in a patient with HIV infection. Indian J Tuberc. 2007;54(4):196-198.

[102] Monno L, Angarano G, Romanelli C, Polymerase chain reaction for non-invasive di-
       agnosis of brain mass lesions caused by Mycobacterium TB: report of five cases in
       human immunodeficiency virus-positive subjects. Tuber Lung Dis 1996;77:280-284

[103] Tandon P. N. Tuberculous meningitis (cranial and spinal) Vinken P. J. and Bruyn G.
       W. (ed.), Handbook of clinical neurology (Elsevier/North Holland Biomedical Press,
       Amsterdam, The Netherlands).1978;33:195-262.

[104] Singh K.K,Nair M.D,Radhakrisnan K,Tyagi J.S. Utility of PCR Assay in Diagnosis of
       En-*Plaque Tuberculoma of* the Brain, J. Clin. Microbiol. 1999; 37(2): 467-47.

[105] Cegielski J.P,Wallace R.J Jr. Infections due to nontuberculous mycobacteria. In:
       Scheld WM, Whitley RJ, Durack DT, eds. Infections of the central nervous system.
       2nd ed. Philadelphia: Lippincott-Raven, 1997:445–461.

[106] Gordon S, Blumber H. Mycobacterium kansasii brain abscess in a patient with AIDS.
       Clin Infect Dis 1992. 14:789–790.

[107] Tandon R, Kye S. Kim, Serrao R. Disseminated Mycobacterium avium-intracellulare
       Infection in a Person With AIDS With Cutaneous and CNS Lesions. The AIDS Read-
       er. 2007 Vol. 17 No. 11.

[108] Fletcher V.P, Schliep T, Schicchi J, Sadr W.E. Central nervous system Mycobacterium
       TB and Mycobacterium avium complex infection in an HIV-positive patient. 14th In-
       ternational AIDS Conference; July 7-12, 2002; Barcelona, Spain. Abstract A10056.

[109] Fortin C. Cerebral Mycobacterium avium abscesses: Late immune reconstitution syn-
       drome in an HIV-1-infected patient receiving highly active antiretroviral therapy.Can
       J Infect Dis Med Microbiol. 2005; 16(3): 187–189.

[110] Murray R, Mallal S, Heath C, French M.Cerebral mycobacterium avium infection in
       an HIV-infected patient following immune reconstitution and cessation of therapy
       for disseminated mycobacterium avium complex infection. Eur J Clin Microbiol In-
       fect Dis. 2001;20(3):199-201. European AIDS Clinical Society guidelines http://
       www.europeanaidsclinicalsociety.org/

[111] Centers for Disease Control and Prevention (CDC). Updated guidelines for the use of
       rifamycins for the treatment of TB among HIV-infected patients taking protease in-
       hibitors or nonnucleoside reverse transcriptase inhibitors. MMWR 2000;49 (No.
       RR-4).

[112] Centers for Disease Control and Prevention (CDC). Prevention and treatment of TB
       among patients infected with human immunodeficiency virus: principles of therapy
       and revised recommendations. MMWR 1998;47:1—58.

[113] American Thoracic Society, CDC, and Infectious Diseases Society of America,June 20,
       2003 / 52(RR11);1-77

[114] Ellard G.A, Humphries M.J, Allen B.W. Cerebrospinal fluid drug concentrations and the treatment of tuberculous meningitis. Am Rev Respir Dis. 1993;148(3):650-655.

[115] Donald P.R.Cerebrospinal fluid concentrations of antiTB agents in adults and children. TB (Edinb). 2010;90(5):279-292

[116] Khushboo J. Nagdev,Rajpal S. Kashyap, Manmohan M. Parida, Rajkumar C. Kapgate, Loop-Mediated Isothermal Amplification for Rapid and Reliable Diagnosis of Tuberculous Meningitis *J. Clin. Microbiol.* 2011; 49 (5): 1861-1865.

[117] Patel K, Xue Ming, Williams PL, Robertson KR,James M, Oleske M. Impact of HAART and CNS-penetrating antiretroviral regimens on HIV encephalopathy among perinatally infected children and adolescents. AIDS. 2009; 10; 23(14): 1893–1901.

[118] Antinori A, Lorenzini P, Giancola LM, Picchi G, Baldini F. Antiretroviral CNS Penetration-Effectiveness (CPE) 2010 ranking predicts CSF viral suppression only in patients with undetectable HIV-1 RNA in plasma,18th CROI, Conference on Retroviruses and Opportunistic Infections Boston, MA.

[119] Shipton L.K, Wester C.W, Stock S. Safety and efficacy of nevirapine- and efavirenz-based antiretroviral treatment in adults treated for TB-HIV co-infection in Botswana. Int J Tuberc Lung Dis. 2009;13(3):360-366.

[120] Friedland G, Khoo S, Jack C, Lalloo U. Administration of efavirenz (600 mg/day) with rifampicin results in highly variable levels but excellent clinical outcomes in patients treated for TB and HIV. J Antimicrob Chemother. Dec 2006;58(6):1299-1302

[121] Centers for Disease Control and Prevention (CDC). Acquired rifamycin resistance in persons with advanced HIV disease being treated for active TB with intermittent rifamycin-based regimens. MMWR 2002;51:214–5.

[122] Vidal J.E, Hernández A.V, Oliveira A.C, de Souza A.L, Madalosso G. Cerebral tuberculomas in AIDS patients: a forgotten diagnosis? Arq Neuropsiquiatr. 2004; 62(3B): 793-796.

[123] Minagar A, Schatz N.J, Glaser J.S. Case report: one-and-a-half-syndrome and TB of the pons in a patient with AIDS. AIDS Patient Care STDS. 2000 Sep;14(9):461-464.

[124] Thonell L, Pendle S, Sacks L. Clinical and Radiological Features of South African Patients with Tuberculomas of the Brain, Clin Infect Dis. 2000; 31 (2): 619-620.

[125] Crump J.A,. Tyrer M.J, Lloyd-Owen S.J, Han L.Y, Lipman M.C, Johnson M.A. Miliary TB with paradoxical expansion of intracranial tuberculomas complicating human immunodeficiency virus infection in a patient receiving highly active antiretroviral therapy. Clin Infect Dis. 1998;26:1008-1009.

[126] Suchindran S, Brouwer E.S, Van Rie A. Is HIV infection a risk factor for multi-drug resistant TB? A systematic review. PLoS One. 2009;4(5):e5561. Epub 2009 May 15

[127] Lukoye D, Cobelens F.G.J, Ezati N, Kirimunda S, Adatu F.E. et al. Rates of Anti-TB Drug Resistance in Kampala-Uganda Are Low and Not Associated with HIV Infection. PLoS ONE 2011;6(1): e16130. doi:10.1371/journal.pone.0016130

[128] Gandhi N.R, Moll A, Sturm A.W, Pawinski R, Govender T, Lalloo U, Zeller K, Andrews J, Friedland G. Extensively drug-resistant TB as a cause of death in patients co-infected with TB and HIV in a rural area of South Africa. Lancet. 2006;368:1575–1580.

[129] Lawn S.D, Bekker L.G, Miller R.F. Immune reconstitution disease associated with mycobacterial infections in HIV-infected individuals receiving antiretrovirals. Lancet Infect Dis; 2005;5:361–373.

[130] Meintjes G, Lawn S.D, Scano F, Maartens G, French M.A, Worodria W, Elliott J.H, Murdoch D.TB-associated immune reconstitution inflammatory syndrome: case definitions for use in resource-limited settings. Lancet Infect Dis. 2008;8(8):516-523.

[131] Shipton L.K, Wester C.W, Stock S, Ndwapi N, Gaolathe T. Safety and efficacy of nevirapine- and efavirenz-based antiretroviral treatment in adults treated for TB-HIV co-infection in Botswana. Int J Tuberc Lung Dis. Mar 2009;13(3):360-366.

[132] Dean G.L, Edwards S.G, Ives N.J, Matthews G, Fox E.F, Navaratne L.Treatment of TB in HIV-infected persons in the era of highly active antiretroviral therapy. AIDS. 2002;16:75–83.

[133] Dheda K, Lampe F.C, Johnson M.A, Lipman M.C. Outcome of HIV-associated TB in the era of highly active antiretroviral therapy. J Infect Dis. 2004;190:1670–1676.

Chapter 2

Tuberculous Pleural Effusion

Wolfgang Frank

Additional information is available at the end of the chapter

1. Introduction

Tuberculosis (TB) has traditionally been one of the major causes of pleural disease and until the earlier decades of the past century held as a principal paradigm of "pleuritis". Indeed in the presence of a distinctly exudative effusion and a compatible clinical presentation the widely used term "pleuritis exudativa" insinuated a tuberculous aetiology and has therefore been understood to be synonymous with "pleuritis exudativa tuberculosa". Whilst in the era of TB decline in the Western hemisphere the term "pleuritis exudativa" (which actually is a tautology!) has largely survived but should now describe exudative effusions in general, the full and precise term "pleuritis exudativa tuberculosa" is therefore suggested whenever the possibility of a tuberculous background is addressed. Otherwise the term "tuberculous pleurisy" or "tuberculous pleuritis" is used to describe this entity, in some countries also the term "specific pleurisy" is common. Apart from acute pleuritis exudative tuberculosa, TB of the pleura may however rarely present as a rather chronic disease state in terms of caseous pleurisy or specific (i. e. tuberculous) empyema, respectively. The following chapter reviews the different features and mechanisms of tuberculous pleural involvement as well as their diagnostic and therapeutic implications.

2. Epidemiology

In many regions of the world tuberculous effusion maintains its role as the leading inflammatory pleural disease. With the worldwide unabated HIV epidemic and related immune deficiency syndrome this state of affairs is likely to continue or being even aggravated within least in certain high risk populations. On a global scale the current significance of human immunodeficiency virus (HIV)-co-infection may be illustrated by WHO data, indicating at a TB-prevalence of 1/3 of the world´s population – similar to the past decade – a HIV-association of approximately 13 % by the year 2009 [1, 2]. Conversely it is assumed, that 33 % to 50 % of HIV infected individuals are co-infected with M. tuberculosis [2]. The MTB/HIV-association however shows a huge intercontinental and regional variance, with the highest rate of HIV-pleural tuberculosis-coincidence being reported in Zimbabwe where 95 % of Patients with tuberculosis pleurisy were HIV positive [3]. In Burundi and Tansania a HIV-coinfection was found in 60 % of all cases of tuberculous pleurisy [4]. One of the lowest rates is reported from Spain with 10 % [5]. Am example of the impact of a high HIV-endemic environment on the incidence of tuberculous pleurisy is also given in a series from Ruanda, where TB accounted for as much as 86 % of all diagnosed pleural effusions [4]. Pleurisy incidence obviously and essentially parallels variability of global TB prevalence with an overwhelming share of 95 % occurring in developing countries. In TB-patients as a whole, pleural involvement varies between ~ 3-5 % in Western Europe and the USA vs. ~ 30 % in developing, HIV-high-preva-lence-countries [6, 7, 8]. The differences clearly underline the modifying role of immunological determinants, stage and severity of the disease, general health status and nutritional factors. The effect of HIV on the occurrence of pleural involvement in a given TB-patient is illustrated by a study reporting a 38 % pleurisy incidence in AIDS-associated TB as compared with 20 % in matched HIV-negative TB patients [5]. On the basis of the presented data according to even conservative WHO estimates the TB-pleurisy incidence throughout the current decade is expected to remain grossly unchanged compared to the past decade, i. e. 18.2 – 62/100.000 in the developing countries vs. 0.42-0.77/100.000 in Western countries [6, 7, 10]. When the epidemiology of pleurisy (or pleural effusion in general) is analysed in terms of the magnitude of TB-contribution, a probably still valid estimate in Western countries is as low as 0.1 – 0.2 % and remains distinctly < 1 % even when referring to pleurisy in a strict sense (i. e. exudates) [11]. By comparison the previously reported percentages of 30-86 % in developing countries are – and remain – indeed dramatically different.

3. Pathophysiology and natural history

3.1. Immunological and microbiological factors

MTB may affect the pleura at different stages of pulmonary or systemic disease and by a number of different mechanisms. Thus pleural involvement occurs in primary, postprimary and reactivated TB alike and is basically believed to arise directly from contiguous macroscopic or microscopic lung lesions or else lymphogenic or hematogenic spread, but probably also via immunogenic mechanisms. Pleuritis exudativa tuberculosa is by far the most common clinical variety and has been classically interpreted as an early delayed-hypersensitivity-type phe-nomenon rather than direct organ involvement [12, 13]. Many clinical observations and experimental findings are in favour of this hypothesis such as:

• its frequent association with known primary infection and a typical 6-12 weeks latency,

• an often striking absence of significant pulmonary or systemic TB-lesions,

• an often culturally negative or paucibacillary effusion [14],

- the sometimes abundant isolation of specifically purified protein derivative (PPD)- protein sensitized T-lymphocytes from pleural fluid [15] and

- more recently the inducible pleurisy in previously PPD-sensitized animals when exposed to intra-pleural mycobacterial protein.

Also the vigorous expression of inflammatory mediators interleukins (IL) like interferon (IFN) γ, IL-1 and IL-8 observed in this model (or conversely their suppression by antilymphocyte serum) support this view [16, 17].

On the other hand there is also strong evidence, that infectious invasion of the pleural space actually occurs at a substantial, albeit variable degree. At thoracoscopy, even with negative fluids studies, extensive inflammatory granuloma formation and fibrin deposits with unexpected abundant mycobacteria recovery are a common finding (see also section on invasive endoscopic-bioptic studies) [18]. The increasingly emerging evidence of a preferred association of TB-pleurisy with reactivated TB in Western populations clearly points to infectious as well as immunological mechanisms being interrelated and operative in a complex manner. Direct infectious invasion however clearly prevails in chronic tuberculous involvement of the pleura as in specific empyema.

According to present views and based on experimental evidence the sequence of immunological processes involved in TB-pleuritis appears to follow a three stage pattern of cellular reactions and granuloma formation as a topic variant of general interaction mechanisms between MTB and the human immune system. A schematic representation is given in figure 1 [19, 20].

Any trigger-mechanism that allows access of mycobacterial protein to the pleura will set off a rapid mesothelial cell initiated and IL-8 mediated polymorphonuclear neutrophil (PMN) influx within a few hours [21]. In addition macrophages and blood-borne monocytes determine this IL-1, IL-6 and tumor necrosis factor (TNF)-α-orchestrated *early stage* reaction.

Within roughly 3 days, in the following *intermediate stage* lymphocyte subpopulations, mainly of CD4+ helper cells but also a substantial CD8+ cytotoxic (natural killer cells) fraction dominate the scene resulting in a CD4+/CD8+-ratio of ~ 4.3 [22]. A minor contribution includes so-called T-cell receptor double negative (DN) $\alpha\beta$-T-cells and $\gamma\delta$-T-cells which appear to have regulatory functions. More recently in tuberculous pleural fluid another unique CD4+CD25+ T-cell-class could be demonstrated being specifically involved in the down-regulation of autoreactive IFN-γ-producing T-cells, thus preventing inflammatory overshoot [23]. IFN-γ a strong promoter of macrophage activation and granuloma formation (together with TNF-α) is the predominant interleukin in this stage. IFN-γ-producing cells have been phenotypically indentified as CDW29+ subpopulation and make up a substantial portion of the granuloma core structure [24].

The *late phase* is characterised by an equilibrated and sustained CD4+/CD8+ cell-based response with continued IFN-γ release and prolonged granuloma formation. Several modulating interleukins are involved in this process such as T-helper-cells (CD4+)-supporting IL-12 and counter-regulatory antiinflammarory cytokines like IL-10 and transforming growth factor (TGF-β).

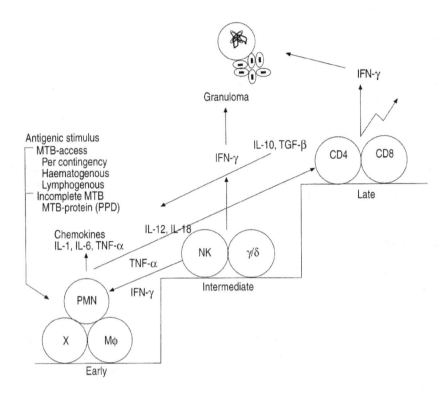

Figure 1. Mechanisms and immunogenesis of tuberculous pleurisy: the three stages of protective immune response. IFN: interferon; TNF: tumor necrosis factor; IL: interleukin; PMN: polymorphonuclear granulocyte; X: undefined cell; MΦ: macrophage, MTB: mycobacterium tuberculosis; PPD purified protein derivative

Results of HIV and AIDS research also emphasize the importance of T-cell response. Several working groups have shown, that the prevalence of tuberculous pleurisy in HIV-infected patients with TB is strikingly correlated with their CD4+ blood lymphocyte count. In one series pleurisy prevalence in individuals with a count of > 200 cells/ml was 27 % as compared to 10 % in those with a count of < 200 cells/ml [25]. The data support the view, that the clinical expression of exudative pleural effusion requires a largely intact cellular immune system and features pleurisy as a high activity response in a still immunocompetent individual. In epidemiologic terms one would conclude that pleural effusion should be more frequent in the still immunocompetent host than in patients with AIDS. In reality however in most HIV-high-prevalence countries like South Africa, Uganda and Zimbabwe the percentage of thoracic TB-patients with pleural effusion is reportedly higher in HIV+ patients [26]. As an explanation the situation is probably blurred by a variable and poorly defined immune status in HIV+ individuals.

3.2. Other factors

The mechanisms of fluid accumulation and of abundant protein leakage to the pleura with often extensive fibrin deposits in tuberculous pleurisy have so far not been fully elucidated. In actual fact pleuritis exudativa tuberculosa generally presents with the highest protein levels commonly seen in exudative conditions. The intensity of inflammation and a proportionately increased vascular permeability would provide a satisfying explanation [25, 27] although at least in animal models, no such significantly altered vascular permeability could be demonstrated [12]. Current opinion holds that grossly impeded lymphatic protein clearance from the pleura due to altered parietal lymphatic channels is probably of tantamount importance.

Again the *entry mechanism* of mycobacteria to the pleura has remained unclear. It is usually assumed that the release of infectious material from a ruptured subpleural TB-lesion is the most common mechanism. While this is likely to occur in more or less extensive pulmonary TB, it would not explain the frequent association of tuberculous pleuritis with an – at least radiographically – unaffected lung. There are also no convincing data yet to quantify the contribution of a purported hematogenous or lymphogenous contribution. One might reasonably speculate that different patterns of pleural tuberculous involvement are operative which might correspond to the different clinical settings of primary, post-primary and reactivated TB.

Caseous tuberculous pleuritis or specific empyema is nowadays a rare condition which is believed to be the result of longstanding or chronic infection of the pleura, when either caseous material gains access to the pleura or chronic pleuritis develops on the background of impaired local defence such as pre-existing fibrous damage of the pleura or as a sequel and complication of artificial pneumothorax, oleothorax or other TB-specific surgery dating back to the pre-chemotherapy era. Correspondingly there is usually an extremely long history often with a remarkable paucity or even absence of symptoms. Penetration to deeper chest wall structures (specific abscess) and ultimately transcutaneous discharge (empyema necessitans) or creation of a specific bronchopleural fistula, as not infrequently seen in the pre-chemotherapeutic era, may complicate this condition [27]. Putrid discharge from a thoracic mass or putrid expectoration with or without haemoptysis may ultimately advert to the condition.

4. Clinical manifestations and natural course

Tuberculous pleurisy may occur as an acute, subacute or rather chronic disease. At times the course is also surprisingly oligosymtomatic. Therefore duration of symptoms or major illness prior to hospital admission and diagnosis varies considerably from < 1 week (31 %) to < 1months (62 %) or even longer (7 %) [28]. These data refer to the pre-HIV era and would not apply for HIV-seropositive patients and elderly populations, which both tend to have a particularly long symptomatic or else oligosymtomatic period. An infectious, i. e. febrile illness is nevertheless by far the most common clinical presentation. As a general rule, an acute febrile illness is the more likely to occur the younger and the more immunocompetent a given patient is. In developing, high-prevalence and high primary-TB-affected countries the age peak of incidence is in the mid thirties, whereas in industrialized countries with a major contribution of reactivated TB it has shifted to about 50 yrs [29]. But still the age-related incidence peak of tuberculous pleuritis is distinctly lower than of parenchymal pulmonary TB which used to peak around 55 yrs [30]. Implicitly by the same statement in Western populations TB-pleurisy was historically more symptomatic than is currently the case. In a representative series from the 1960-1970s ~ 60 % of patients developed an acute illness mimicking bacterial (pleuro)-pneumonia with cough (70 %), chest pain (75 %) and low- to high-grade fever (86 %) as the most frequent symptoms [31, 32]. Other symptoms include those commonly occurring in various TB disease states such as weight loss, malaise and night sweat. Severe or even live threatening disease, defined as persistent high-grade fever > 38,3°C over > 2 weeks or respiratory distress has been in reported in a more recent series in only 7 % [31], whereas an oligosymptomatic or a febrile course is described in 14-33 % [32]. Tuberculous pleurisy usually involves one hemithorax only (90-95 %) and is of limited size (roughly up to one-half of the hemithorax volume). In a major series (n=254) effusions occupying more than 2/3 of a hemithorax were noted in only 18 % [33]. Rarely effusion will occupy the entire hemithorax and will almost never reveal compressive or displacing features [31]. Basically there are no specific clinical clues to tuberculous etiology in pleurisy unless some TB-contact is revealed or suspected. An HIV-related background may be suspected in a compatible clinical and history setting or when there is a long preclinical period, unusual additional symptoms like diarrhea and more hepato(spleno)-megaly or lymphadenopathy as might be attributed to the tuberculous condition. Untreated, lone pleuritis exudativa tuberculosa in the short term seems to be a self-limited inflammatory process in most instances, terminating in complete or incomplete resolution within weeks or month. Frequently observed otherwise unexplained diaphragmatic adhesions may be a late sequel of clinical silent or oligosymtomatic TB pleurisy. Importantly however progression or reactivation to active pleuropulmonary or extrapulmonary TB occurs in an important fraction. In one follow-up study the recurrence rate within 1 year was 5 %, where TB did not relapse earlier than 8 month after the onset of pleurisy. Within a 4-5 yr period however the rate was dramatically higher and in initially culture positive and culture negative subjects with 65 % and 60 % respectively roughly alike [27]. One major outcome determinant clearly is the presence and the extent of pulmonary involvement. At a similar therapeutic intensity in a very recent major clinical study from Taiwan, 51 (24,9 %) out of 205 hospitalised patients having been identified to have isolated (lone) pleuritis had a significantly better outcome, shorter hospital stay and less comorbidity than the patients with pleuropulmonary disease [34].

5. Diagnosis

5.1. Clinical findings

5.1.1. Signs at physical examination

Physical examination clearly will provide only non-specific signs of pleural effusion in general including dullness to percussion and the occasional demonstration of a pleural rub at auscultation ("snow-ball-crunching sign") in particular in the presence of chest pain. Signs of a trapped or loculated rather than free flowing fluid collection may suggest a tuberculous aetiology, but this observation holds also true for "plain" parapneumonic pleurisy. Usual signs of systemic infection, as mentioned above, that should be looked for, may alert to the possibility of a HIV-related background.

5.1.2. Imaging studies

Imaging techniques are engaged in the evaluation of tuberculous pleurisy following general diagnostic pathway recommendations for effusion. *Conventional chest radiography (CRX)* requires fluid amounts of at least 150 ml to become clearly detectable as blunting of the costodiaphragmatic angle in standard projections. Profuse effusion with opacification of an entire hemithorax would rather favour differential diagnoses like malignancy in the elderly and afebrile patient [35]. Free flowing effusion may be easily identified, but one should look specifically for signs of loculation, pleural thickening or adhesions and in profuse effusion for compressive signs interfering with the respiratory performance. Apart from pleural changes pulmonary infiltrates, nodules, lymphnodes and other suggestive signs of TB like encapsulated or cavitary lesions must be carefully looked for using routine *CT-imaging.* CT-based prevalence of lung perenchymal tuberculous lesions in mixed populations appears to be significantly higher than previously assessed based on conventional radiography. In one recent series from Korea comprising 106 patients with an age distribution from 16-89 yrs (mean 53) with 86% a remarkable high rate of parenchymal changes was found, presumed to represent active tuberculosis in 59 % [36]. Most of these lesions revealed features of reactivated rather than primary tuberculosis. *Sonography (Ultrasound, US)* using innovative technical achievements like high frequency (5-7.5 MHz) – US and convex or sector scanners allow extended exploration of the chest wall structures, the diaphragm and the anterior mediastinum up to a penetration depth of ~ 25 cm. Specific advantages of US are a more precise fluid volumetry than by CRX, precise localisation of septae, membranes and chambers as well as pleural thickening along with its particular versatility for bedside diagnosis. On demand guidance for interventions such as thoracentesis is a particular asset of US.. Examples are shown in figure 2, 3. *Magnetic-resonance imaging (MRI)* is a highly refined, not generally available technique, which will rarely be required but does have differential diagnostic merits in the analysis of critical borderline relationships i. e. distinguishing between inflammatory-infiltrative and malignant-destructive pleural processes via different T-weighted sequences [37]. Very recently a role of PET-CT has also been described. PET-imaging may indeed provide differently extensive focal and impressing laminar changes which however remain indistinguishable from malignant lesions [38].

5.2. Immunologic tests

5.2.1. Tuberculin skin reaction

The tuberculin skin reaction is traditionally considered an indispensable tool in the diagnosis of tuberculosis in general and likewise in tuberculous pleurisy although it is less reliable than in pulmonary TB. The rate of false negative reactions to PPD has been given as high 30 % of cases but even figures up to < 41 % have been reported [31, 32, 33], the variability possibly reflecting non-standardised test doses. Still however there remains an amazing false negative rate. There is no absolutely satisfying hypothesis to explain this paradoxon, let alone unequiv-

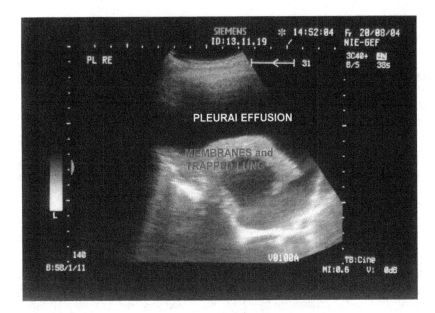

Figure 2. Ultrasound detection of inflammatory visceral membranes and consecutively trapped lung in pleuritis exudativa tuberculosa

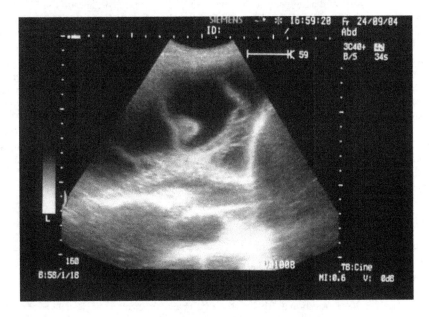

Figure 3. Ultrasound detection of multiple chambers in pleuritis exudativa tuberculosa

ocal experimental evidence. It appears a valid speculation to consider a local pooling of sensitised T-lymphocytes at the site of infection responsible. Animal experiments and clinical investigations have shown sequestration of PPD-sensitized lymphocytes to the pleural compartment actually to occur in the early phase of infection leading to their systemic depletion [39]. As a presumptive additional mechanism the presence of adhering suppressor cells to blood lymphocytes has been demonstrated in PPD-anergic patients [39]. While the explanatory evidence may remain scanty, it should be emphasised that in clinical practice the phenomenon appears to be transitory and restricted to the early phase of tuberculous infection. It might thus be associated with the pre-allergic phase of tuberculous infection, since conversion of skin reactivity has been subsequently observed within a 6-8 weeks delay [27]. As a reverse conclusion in the framework of discussed hypotheses the observation of a delayed PPD-conversion might be interpreted as a clue to primary infection to have occurred. Persisting anergy would then point to other immune-modulating factors like advanced age, certain drug interference or immune-compromising comorbidity.

5.2.2. Interferon-γ-release assays

In Europe commercially available Interferon-γ-release assays (IGRA) are the QuantiFERON-TB-Gold-Test and the T-Spot-TB-Test. Both use the MTB-RD1-region antigen sequences CFP10 and ESAT 6 and measure the specific lymphocyte-induced quantitative IFN-γ-response or the sensitized IFN-γ-producing lymphocyte response, respectively. There has been elaborated a body of clinical data in practical use highlighting both the assets and pitfalls of the investigation. In summary and in general there is distinct superiority to the PPD-skin-test with an overall sensitivity of ~ 85 % and a high specificity well > 90 % [40]. The concordance of the PPD-test and IFN-γ-release assays is in the order of 60-85 % [41]. However in the identification of active clinical tuberculosis blood-based IFN-γ-release assays also have revealed a considerable rate of false negative findings. In several studies including pulmonary a well as pleural tuberculosis, sensitivity was limited to 60-64 % [42, 43, 44]. There have also been a number of inconsistent and equivocal reports where the results obviously vary with different TB-prevalence settings (i. e. pretest probability). In a number of studies the variability of sensitivity ranges between 96 % in low prevalence settings down to 58 % in studies featuring high prevalence areas, also specificity setbacks are reported [45]. Blood-based IGRA´s therefore seem to share the limitations of PPD-testing. Since they cannot distinguish latent from active TB, in conclusion, the diagnostic value for identification of tuberculous pleurisy in high prevalence settings is very low and has even only limited value in industrialized countries.

5.3. Pleural fluid analysis

5.3.1. Biochemical parameters

When there is enough effusion to allow safe puncture and TB is suspected, *thoracentesis* is a mandatory diagnostic step. The effusion will be invariably and markedly exudative with a (unless in tuberculous empyema) clear, straw- to amber-coloured appearance and a mean protein content above 5.0 g/dl, in one series (n=83) it was 5.2 g/dl (range 3.5 – 7.0) [32]. Glucose and pH-values have traditionally believed to be characteristically low in TB. It appears however, that on the basis of more recent data, as also confirmed in the author´s own experience these values are not substantially different from exudates due to other aetiologies. SAHN [46] found pH-values < 7.29 and glucose values < 30 mg/dl in only 20% of patients and this has been confirmed by others [47]. Interestingly however, if low values actually occur, they appear to correlate with the pleural bacillary load and are to some extent predictive of cultural results. In one thoracoscopic study positive pleural fluid culture yield was 59 % when the glucose level was < 50 mg/dl but only 25 % when the glucose values were > 50 mg/dl (p<0.005) [18]. Lactic dehydrogenase (LDH) is a non-specific marker of pleural inflammation, which may be excessively elevated in tuberculous pleurisy, although with a mean value of 423 IU/ml (range 43 – 1.575) as reported in a representative series again does not discriminate TB from para-pneumonic and not even from malignant effusion [32]. Adenosine deaminase (ADA) has been a promising and much hailed semispecific biochemical parameter. ADA is an inflammatory enzyme expressed predominantly by sensitized and activated T-lymphocytes. Isoenzymes (ADA2) in addition reflect to some extent monocyte/macrophage activation. Thus increased ADA-activity in general indicates various T cell/macrophage interactive inflammatory processes like granulomatous disease but also empyema and collagen vascular disease. It appears however particularly sensitive to TB. In a key study (n=129) in patients < 35 yrs a receiver operating characteristics (ROC) –derived cut-off level of 47 U/ml allowed distinction of tuberculous effusion from empyema, rheumatic and neoplastic disease with a 100 % sensitivity and 87.5 specificity. When empyema was eliminated, specificity and the positive predictive value even attained 100 % [48]. There are important limitations to the interpretation of these results and their clinical relevance:

- the data reflect the afore mentioned age group only, in more heterogenous groups both sensitivity and specificity have to be (down)-corrected to 95 % and 90 % respectively [22, 49, 50].

- the results strictly apply to high TB prevalence settings only and do not allow for different pre-test probabilities [3].

- also immune suppression like in AIDS endemic areas may interfere with inflammatory ADA-release and invalidate diagnostic conclusions [3, 51].

Nevertheless, based on the most accepted cut-off level of 40 IU/l and provided its critical use in areas of at least intermediate TB-prevalence ADA determination must be regarded as a true diagnostic enrichment. An era of successful ADA-use has been recently summarized and confirmed by a large size metaanalysis (63 studies, 5297 tuberculous and non-tuberculous effusions) resulting in a sensitivity and specificity of 92 % and 90 % respectively [52].

5.3.2. Cytological analysis

Based on the immunological processes involved, a marked lymphocytosis is the predicted and characteristic feature of TB-pleurisy along with significantly increased total white cell counts as reflected in one representative study with a mean count of 2.309/mm^3 (range 30 – 24.009 mm^3) [32]. Usually 90 – 95 % of pleural fluid cells are T-lymphocytes, the remainder being B-lymphocytes and (mostly) activated mesothelial cells. Only exceptionally (in ~ 5 %) lympho-cyte counts < 50 % may occur [27]. Thus when an 80 % lymphocyte reference line is chosen, pleuritis tuberculosa exudativa is by far the most frequent cause of pleural lymphocytosis [46]. Rarely, in particular in the early phase of inflammation fluid cytology may reveal neutrophil leucocyte (PMN) predominance. Expansion of the eosinophil compartment would be an extremely unusual finding. In the presence of significant numbers of eosinophils (> 5 %) differential diagnoses should be considered.

5.3.3. Microbiological studies

The microbiological yield from diagnostic (low volume) thoracentesis as far the smear is concerned is very low unless the whole effusion or large amounts are being centrifuged or the patient has a tuberculous empyema [14, 29]. In HIV positive individuals, particularly in those with CD4 cell counts < 200 x 10^6/l significantly higher yields are being reported amounting in one study to 37 % vs. 0 % in non HIV-patients [53]. In a comprehensive study on microbiologic smear findings in pleural fluid specimens in non-selected HIV negative out-patients, the positive acid fast smear yield (n=232) again was actually zero [54]. Cultures should be obtained both from the sputum and pleural fluid. The positive cultural yield from pleural fluid has been given in collective reviews with 10 – 35 %, being ~ 25 % in the mean [14, 30]. In one of the largest series (n=100] the sensitivity of pleural fluid culture was 28 % [18, 55]. The use of radiometric or non-radiometric liquid culture systems (BACTEC, MB/BacT, MGIT) will markedly accelerate results and possibly lead to an enhanced yield (~ 50 %), when bedside instead of laboratory inoculation is used [56]. The yield of sputum cultures in tuberculous effusion is expectedly largely dependent on the extent and nature of pulmonary involvement and may mount up to ~ 50 %. In the non-expectorating patient the use of induced sputum is advised [57]. The positive yield is also believed to be higher in HIV-infected patients [53, 57]. In the complete absence of pulmonary lesions according to most sources the sensitivity will be no more than 4-7 % [30]. Only exceptionally a surprisingly high figure of 31 % for induced sputum has been reported [57].

5.3.4. Immunological and molecular studies

Immunological studies of pleural fluid in TB-pleurisy focus on the measurement and analysis of chemokins and interleukins that are characteristically associated with the tuberculous immune response. TNFα and IFNγ revealed at a cut-off 140 pg/ml a sensitivity of 94 % and a specificity of 85 % [58,60]. Similarly as for ADA the major confounders were bacterial empyema and parapneumonic effusion respectively. Interestingly TNFα did not attain enough discriminatory power to separate TB from various inflammatory conditions and is no more considered a valid option in the diagnosis of TB. More recent meta analysis-derived collective data from 22 studies resulted in an overall sensitivity of 89 % at a 97 % specificity [61]. Thus at present IFNγ-determination in pleural fluid – contrasting to systemic IGRA-application – would appear a useful diagnostic test with a sensitivity and discriminatory power comparable to that of ADA-determination if one was to accept the significantly higher costs and disregard more powerful diagnostic options as provided by subsequently discussed invasive biopsy techniques.

Molecular mycobacterial identification methods employing a variety of *nucleic acid amplifica-tion techniques (NAAT)* have been applied in TB pleurisy with considerable enthusiasm and expectations ever since their first application in TB in 1989 [62]. The techniques that have been used include target amplification (polymerase chain reaction, PCR), strand displacement amplification (SDA), transcription mediated amplification (TMA), probe/primer amplification (ligand chain reaction, LCR) and Q-Beta replicase amplification mostly with the IS 6110, 16S recombinant ribonucleic acid (rRNA) and 65 XD target sequence [63-66]. So far published data, both biopsy- and pleural fluid-based have shown considerable variance of diagnostic yield, which ranged from 20-81 % as to sensitivity with an expectedly high specificity in the order of 98-100 % (table 1). When analyzing the sources of this high variance, apart from technical factors like contamination-related "carry over" or amplification inhibitors, the most important determinant appeared to be the number of bacilli in the pleura fluid or specimen sample [31]. Although theoretically requiring the presence of merely one microorganism to trigger amplification, similar to sputum anlysis, failed to detect pleural MTB in particular when the pleurisy was paucibacillar, correlating with cultural negativity. In addition to fluid samples numerous studies have evaluated the value of various nucleic acid extraction and amplifica-tions techniques in formalin-fixed and paraffin-embedded pleural tissue specimen [67-71]. With the use of commercial kits of both DNA amplicons (ligand chain MTB assay, LCxMTB or AMPLICOR MTB) or RNA amplicons (amplified MTB direct test, AMTDT) according to the latest currently available sources, the sensitivity of each single technique did not exceed 63.2 % albeit at an expected 100 % specificity [71]. The so far largest meta-analysis including 40 studies and featuring commercial as well as in-house ("home-brew") tests, confirms a low and heterogeneous sensitivity (in the mean 62 %) and high specificity of 98 % [72]. Thus there is no convincing evidence, that generally and especially in the critical issue of paucibacillar (cultural negative) pleurisy, NAATs perform substantially better in tissue than in effusion specimens (table 1). Although in-house assays have been reported to be slightly superior [73], there remain significant sensitivity set backs both in liquid- and tissue-derived specimen. In summary NAATs may offer certain advantages like quick results within hours or added specificity. They may also improve sensitivity in combined and parallel use with conventional methods and multiple amplicors (diagnostic confirmation), but can certainly not replace or obviate the need for conventional tools in the diagnosis of TB pleurisy.

5.3.5. Invasive bioptic and endoscopic studies

Bioptic techniques in the evaluation of tuberculous effusions incorporate closed blind or imaging guided needle biopsy and medical (video)-thoracoscopy. Only exceptionally, if ever, surgical diagnostic efforts including video-assisted surgical thoracoscopy (VATS) would appear appropriate. Invasive techniques are indicated when clinical investigation and pleural fluid analysis provide only ambiguous or conflicting results and this is particularly true if relevant differential diagnoses like malignancy need to be reliably excluded. *Needle biopsy* may be considered a first step. There are no clear preferences as to the type of needle to be used, although in the author's opinion the Tru-Cut or Raja-system may be preferable to the older Abrams- or Ramel-needle by providing a larger specimen along with easier han-dling. It is recommended, that at least six biopsies are obtained, since they will not regular-

First Author	case-# TB / non-TB	Amplicor Kit	Sensitivity [%]			Speci-ficity [%]
			overall	culture-positive	culture-negative	
effus.-based						
deWit	53/31	336 r.squ.	81	-	-	78
Lassence	14/10	IS 6110	60	100	50	100
		65 XD	20	66	8	100
Querol	21/86	IS 6110	81	100	60	98
tissue-based						
Salian	25/ 35	IS 6110	73	-	-	100
Marchetti	26/ 11	IS 6110	80-87	100	73-82	100
Gamboa	67/ 97	AMTDT	83	-	-	100
Palacios	18/168	LCxMTB	90.4	-	-	98.5
Ruiz-Manzano	57/ 17	AMTDT/	80.7	-	-	100
		LCxMTB		-	-	100
Pai (eff + tiss)	metaan	various	63.2	-	-	100

Table 1. Role of Nucleic-Acid-Amplification-Techniques (NAAT) in the Diagnosis of Tuberculous Pleuritis

ly contain a representative parietal pleural sample [74]. With this premise and the expected yield of at least two valid samples closed needle biopsy should be diagnostic in tubercu- lous pleurisy in ~ 60 % of cases, when histology and tissue-, as well as fluid-culture are being combined. In a major series (n=100 %) a 61 % positive yield was composed of 51 % biopsy yield and 28 % positive fluid culture (figure 4) [18, 55]. Distinctly higher yields have also been reported in the literature, leading in a collective review to an average sensitivity of 69 % (range 28-88 %) [75]. The difference and wide range is likely to be due to technical disparities and inclusion of data originating from largely different prevalence areas. In one study from a high prevalence area (South Africa) comprising 51 patients with undiagnosed pleurisy the positive closed needle yield in tuberculous pleurisy (histology+AFB-stain+culture) was 79%, when combined with pleural fluid ADA-determination and a lymphocyte/neutrophil ratio > 0.75 sensitivity increased to 93% at a specificity of 100% [76]. Thus with the parallel use of less invasive parameters needle biopsy approaches the diagnostic potency of more inva- sive techniques and would appear the second best diagnostic option in areas with limited medical logistics and resources.

Medical thoracoscopy as a *"window to the pleural space"* [77] is the gold standard procedure in the evaluation of exudative pleural effusion, hence also pleural pleurisy. The current and future role of thoracoscopy needs to be redefined for its diagnostic and interventional efficacy in the light of its close historical affiliation with TB. In fact tuberculosis was already a major focus of medical thoracoscopy or *"pleuroscopy"* as referred to and initiated by JACOBAEUS back in

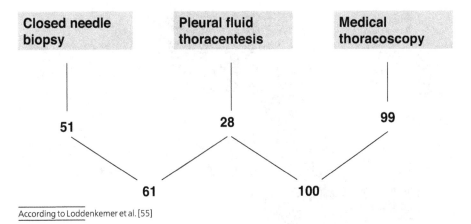

According to Loddenkemer et al. [55]

Figure 4. Single and cumulated yield (%) of various microbiological and bioptical investigations in tuberculous pleurisy

1910 [78]. Anticipating modern minimally invasive surgical techniques, now all included under the heading *video-assisted thoracic surgery (VATS)*, his pioneering approach to thoraco-scopy was basically interventional with the intention to optimize pneumolysis and to break strands for artificial pneumothorax induction in pulmonary TB *("Jacobaeus operation")*. However the ability to visualize major portions of the pleural surface, to intervene in the presence of membranes, adhesions and septae with the option of numerous dedicated biopsies also ensures optimum diagnostic results that are reflected in a yield of 94-99 % as confirmed in decades of clinical experience [18, 77-81]. At thoracoscopy tuberculous pleurisy usually appeals to the experienced investigator with characteristic and fairly diagnostic inflammatory patterns.

- One may present with abundant fibrinous membranes, septae, loculations and diffuse inflammatory thickening of the parietal and visceral pleura as the prevailing pattern. An example of this endoscopic pattern is shown in figure 5.

- A second characteristic feature is a more or less intensive seeding of the pleural surface with solid or caseous, sago-like nodules and only scanty fibrin deposits as shown in figure 6. Although usually fairly small, major nodules as also shown in figure 6 may easily be confused with malignant lesions.

- *Tuberculous empyema* as exemplified in figure 7 may be visually indistinguishable from non-specific bacterial empyema unless calcifications, irreversible lung trapping or suspect pulmonary lesions suggest a tuberculous origin.

Similarly to closed needle biopsy a sufficient number of biopsies – at least three- should be obtained to warrant optimum and representative results. This may often require mechanical debridement of membranes and septae to gain access to the inflamed pleura. When thoraco-

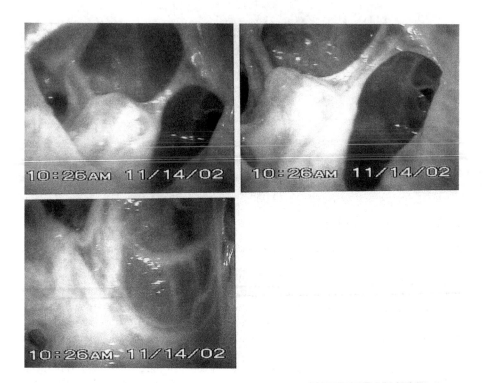

Male 48 years, pleuritis tuberculosa exsudativa

Figure 5. Typical thoracoscopic aspect of fibrin-type multi-loculated effusion including septae and chambers in tuberculous pleurisy

scopic results are combined with aforementioned techniques positive results may be augmented to virtually 100 % (fig. 2) [18].

Thoracoscopy also provides a number of additional advantages:

• With the reasonable diagnostic certainty of visual findings combined with an immediate histological yield of > 90 % it allows instant implementation of antituberculous chemotherapy

• The percentage of positive TB-cultures obtained from biopsies and fibrous membranes may be twice as high (78 %) as from needle biopsies and pleural fluid combined (39 %) [77]. This in turn provides superior opportunity for drug susceptibility testing.

• Complete removal and subsequent drainage of pleural fluid with pulmonary re-expansion provides instant relief to the patients and warrants better healing and outcome options (see section on therapy).

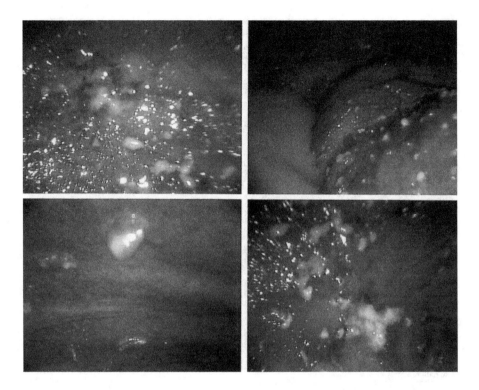

Male 24 years, pleuritis exsudativa tuberculosa

Figure 6. Typical thoracoscopic aspect of sago-type disseminated small and larger nodules both of the parietal and visceral pleura giving rise to confusion with malignancy

- In addition thoracoscopy may be easily expanded to an adjuvant therapeutic intervention by breaking adhesions and debridement of membranes as also discussed in the section on therapy.

In the overall assessment of biopsy techniques the experienced investigator will therefore bypass closed needle biopsy and prefer thoracoscopy. Closed needle biopsy however will remain the second best alternative if

- there is no logistic option for thoracoscopy or

- in the presence of clinical obstacles such as contraindications or mal-detachment of the lung due to adhesions or advanced obliteration of the pleural space.

In summary, for the diagnosis of tuberculous pleurisy it appears and remains a well-founded clinical policy to push for the recovery of biopsy specimens whenever possible and to combine these with less invasive test results to ensure optimum management of the condition.

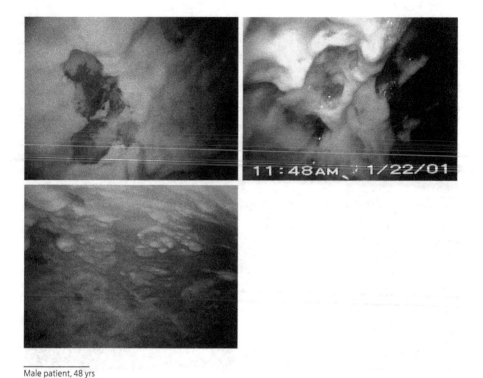

Male patient, 48 yrs

Figure 7. Typical thoracoscopic aspect of tuberculous („specific") empyema showing putrid parietal coverings including bioptic lesion and circumscript coin-like pleural thickening

6. Therapy options

6.1. Systemic therapy

Basically systemic therapy of tuberculous pleurisy in the moderately ill patient neither differs in intensity nor duration from antituberculous chemotherapy of pulmonary and other organ tuberculosis in general. Current short term recommendations for non-complicated pulmonary and extrapulmonary organ tuberculosis call for a quadruple drug therapy in the 2-month acute phase in the combination of 5 mg/kg Isoniacid (INH), 10 mg/kg Rifampicin (RMP), 30-35 mg/kg Pyrazinamid (PZA) and 20-25 mg/kg Ethambutol (EMB) or 15 mg/kg Streptomycin (SM), where daily alternation of the SM and EMB component may be preferable [82]. In the second 4-month stabilizing phase a INH/RMP dual therapy is recommended. Until the 1990-years a triple therapy in the initial phase for Tb was considered safe enough in view of a low incidence of primary drug resistance. The quadruple therapy recommendation is therefore an amendment to a meanwhile globally changed drug susceptibility situation. Thus in an un-clarified clinical setting the extent of drug resistance expectation will modify treatment strategies. The current policy in the case of tuberculous pleurisy therefore holds, that in lone and paucibacillar pleurisy (without lung parenchymal lesions) after immediate quadruple therapy a down-grading to a historical triple scheme is safe enough, provided full drug susceptibility is warranted. In the presence of lung parenchymal involvement the full standard scheme would however apply. The current average drug resistance probability is reflected in one major series (n=78) with a rate of 6.4 %, being probably representative for Middle Europe [55].

The addition of an oral or parenteral steroid regimen to antituberculous drug therapy has been discussed controversially. The rationale put forward for this approach focuses on

• the assumption of a shorter, attenuated clinical course in the severely ill patient,

• improved outcome by prevention of sequels in terms of pulmonary encasement and fibrothorax.

Three valid clinical studies employing a randomized, double-blind controlled design may be considered to have basically settled the issue [83, 84, 85]. These studies consistently showed, that a tapering steroid therapy for 4 and up to 12 weeks starting with 0.5, 0.75 and 1.0 mg/kg/day prednisone added to a standard antituberculous drug regimen, although mitigating and shortening the clinical course to a moderate extent in two studies, did not alter any of the outcome endpoints (clinical status, effusion resolution, pleural sequelae, lung volume and gas exchange). In conclusion from these data, steroids would generally not appear indicated in TB-pleurisy, a reasonable practice however would be a temporary use in the presence of a severe febrile and consumptive clinical course. Their long term use for the prevention of fibrotic sequels would appear obsolete.

6.2. Local therapy

Local therapy is an option, which is usually directly derived from a thoracoscopic approach to the management of the condition. First of all it needs to be emphasized that the (possibly complete) evacuation of pleural effusion is already an important topic treatment approach. While this can basically be achieved by non-endoscopic techniques like simple thoracentesis and small bore catheters as well, there is no doubt, that thoracoscopy will be disparately more effective due to the ability of visual guided optimum positioning and the use of large bore drains. In addition there is ample clinical evidence, that expert medical thoracoscopy can open intrapleural loculations and chambers, completely evacuate sequestrated effusion compartments and also to some extent produce effective debridement of membranes. Although no controlled study has so far proven the value of such efforts, from the view of the expert endoscopist it would appear a straightforward and convincing approach. Together with the early induction of antituberculous chemotherapy it might be responsible for the fact that in our institution over more than two decades of experience none of the patients needed decortication subsequently.

Another more recently discussed approach in topical therapy would be, by a rationale analogue to non-specific bacterial empyema, the use of fibrinolysis (streptokinase) which even need not necessarily be linked to an endoscopic protocol. There is so far only scanty experience [85]. However one fairly comprehensive study from Taiwan using a non-endoscopic pigtail catheter technique and comparing a loculated streptokinase group (n=22) with a loculated normal saline irrigation group (n=22), reported significantly better outcome both in clinical terms of imaging and functional criteria [86]. Additional future evidence provided, this would seem an encouraging step towards further improvement in acute tuberculous pleurisy management.

Surgery in the era of antituberculous chemotherapy is only exceptionally required in the management of tuberculous involvement of the pleura. Remaining indications refer to rare instances of previously mentioned tuberculous empyema and in particular its complications. Specific issues in this context would be excessive membrane formation with trapped lung and significant long term pulmonary encasement due to fibrothorax. Due to the scarcity of pertinent cases and studies (at least in the western hemisphere) there are no generally accepted surgical guidelines for the management of these conditions. Surgical decisions must be created in an individual case-determined approach. A reasonable policy would appear to perform lone or combined empyemectomy/pleurectomy, also termed *early decortication* in clinically severe and functionally disabling conditions refractory to medical efforts. These indications may be amenable to video-assisted thoracic surgery (VATS)-based interventions. Formal thoracotomy would however be required if it comes to additional lung parenchymal resection or thoraco-plasty in rare complicated cases e.g. with persisting pyopneumothorax with or without trapped lung due to a large, medically intractable broncho-pleural fistula.

A different issue is severe, chronically trapped lung due to fibrothorax. A reserved approach to surgical strategies is generally advised because unexpected long term remission of inflammatory peels is sometimes impressing. Although decortication has been performed as early as 6 weeks after the precipitating insult (empyema), the indication to *late decortication* is basically dis-cussed in the context of definitely and irreversibly trapped lung (fibrothorax) i.e. when at least 6 months have elapsed. With a focus on repair of lung function and prevention of chest deformity most investigators agree that the indication requires a significant decrement of lung function (TLC<60% pred., reduction of perfusion>50%) and level of deformity in the absence of significant calcifications (*pleuritis calcarea*). Even then with extensive fibrotic fusion of both pleural sheaths not only will surgery be fraught with considerable technical problems but also the certainty and extent of functional improvement may not be predictable and warranted.

6.3. Sequels and prognosis

There are largely diverging data as to the prevalence of fibrothorax and permanent pleural thickening as the most important sequel of pleural TB. In one source based on standard radiographs in pleuritis exudative tuberculosa a percentage as high as 49 % has been given [32]. With the strict definition of fibrothorax as a pleural membrane of at least 5 mm thickness extending across major portions of the hemithorax and persisting > 8 weeks after initiation of therapy a figure of ~ 5 % is a more likely and widely accepted rate of this complication. The intensity of pleural inflammation expressed as interleukin levels and derangement of bio-chemical parameters is assumed to be to some extent predictive for this complication. In one study residual pleural thickening was indeed significantly correlated with the magnitude of the intitial change of inflammatory glucose-, pH- and TNF-α-levels [87].

Caseous tubercus pleurisy and specific empyema respectively is in its natural course and in prognostic terms an entirely different entity. These patients will invariably and typically develop an extensive calcified fibrothorax (pleuritis calcarea) with or without concomitant chest deformity. Also chronic non-specific lung disease (COPD) with or without bronchiectasis, late TB-exacerbations and internal or external fistulisation (specific empyema necessitans) may develop. Anecdotical occurrence of non-HODGKIN lymphomas arising from long term smouldering encasements has also been described.

Author details

Wolfgang Frank*

Address all correspondence to: wfrank@klinikamsee.de

Lungenklinik Amsee, Waren (Müritz), Germany

References

[1] Dolin, P. J, Raviglione, M. C, & Kochi, A. Global tuberculosis incidence and mortality during (1990). Bull WHO 1994; , 72, 213-220.

[2] Tomford JW wwwclevelandclinicmeded.com (2010).

[3] Riantawan, P, Chaowalit, P, Wongsangeiem, M, & Rojanaraweewong, P. Diagnostic value of pleural fluid adenosine deaminase in tuberculous pleuritis with reference to HI coinfection and a Bayesian analysis Chest (1999). , 116, 97-103.

[4] Batungwanayo, J, Taelman, H, Allen, S, et al. Pleural effusion, tuberculosis and HIV-1 infection in Kigali, Rwanda AIDS (1993). , 7, 73-79.

[5] Luzze, H, Elliott, A. M, Joloba, M. L, et al. Evaluation of suspected tuberculous pleurisy: clinical and diagnostic findings in HIV-positive and HIV-negative adults in Uganda Internat J Tub Lung Dis (2001). , 5, 746-753.

[6] Seibert, A. F, Haynes, J, & Middleton, R. Bass JB Tuberculous pleural effusion: twenty years experience Chest (1991). , 99, 883-886.

[7] Mlika-cabanne, N, Brauner, M, Magusi, F, et al. Radiographic abnormalities in tuberculosis and coexisting human immunodeficiency virus infection: results from Dares Salaam, Tanzania Am Rev Respir Crit Care Med (1995). , 152, 786-793.

[8] Saks, A. M, & Posner, R. Tuberculosis in HIV positiv patients in South Africa; A comparative radiological study with HIV negative patients Clin Radiol (1992). , 46, 387-390.

[9] Perez-Rodriguez, E, & Jimenez, D. Light RW Effusions from tuberculosis In: Light RW, Gary Lee YC eds. Textbook of Pleural Disease Arnold, (2003). , 329.

[10] Mehta, J. B, Dutt, A, & Harvill, L. Matthews KM Epidemiology of extrapulmonary tuberculosis Chest (1991).

[11] Light RW Approach to the patient In: Light RWed. Pleural Disease 3rd edn. Baltimore Williams and Wilinson (1995).

[12] Allen, J. C. Apicella MA Experimental pleural effusion as a manifestation of delayed hypersensivity to tuberculin PPD J Immunol (1968). , 101, 481-487.

[13] Yamamoto, S, & Dunn, C. J. Wolloughby DA Studies on delayed hypersensitivity to pleural exudates in guinea pigs: II. The interrelationship of monocytic and lymphocytic cells with respect to migration activity Immunology (1976). , 30, 513-519.

[14] Bueno, C. E, Clemente, G, Castro, B. C, et al. Cytologic and bacteriologic analysis of fluid and pleural biopsy specimens with Copes needle Arch Intern Med (1990). , 1190-1194.

[15] Fujiwara, H, & Tsuyuguchi, I. Frequency of tuberculine reactive T-lymphocytes in pleural fluid and blood from patients with tuberculous pleurisy Chest (1986). , 89, 530-532.

[16] Leibowitz, S, & Kennedy, L. Lessof MH The tuberculin reaction in the pleural cavity and its suppression by antilymphocyte serum Br J Exp Pathol (1973). , 54, 481-487.

[17] Antony, V. B, Sahn, S. A, & Antony, A. C. Repine JE Bacillus Calmette-Guerin-stimulated neutrophils release chemotaxins for monocytes in rabbit pleural space in vitro Clin Invest (1985). , 76, 1414-1421.

[18] Loddenkemper, R, & Boutin, C. Thoracoscopy: Diagnostic and therapeutic Indications Eur Respir J (1993). , 6, 1544-1555.

[19] Kaufmann SHEKaplan G. Immunity to intracellular bacteria Editorial Overview Res Immunol (1996). , 487.

[20] Schluger, N. W. Rom WL The host immune response to tuberculosis. State of the Art Am J Respir Crit Care Med (1998). , 157, 679-691.

[21] Antony, V. B, Hott, J. W, Kunkel, S. L, et al. Pleural mesothelial cell expression ov C-C (monocyte chemotactic peptide) and C-X-C (interleukin 8] chemokines Am J Respir Cell Mol Biol (1995). , 12, 5812-588.

[22] Fontes Baganha MPego A., Lima MA et al. Serum and pleural adenosine deaminase: correlation with lymphocytic populations. Chest (1990). , 97, 605-610.

[23] Qin, X. J, Shi, H. Z, Liang, Q. I, et al. CD4+CD25+ regulatory T lymphocytes in tuberculous pleural effusion Chin Med J (2008). , 581-586.

[24] Barnes, P. F, Mistry, S. D, Cooper, C. L, et al. Compartimentalization of a CD4 T-lymphocyte subpopulation in tuberculous pleural effusions J Immunol (1989). , 142, 1114-1119.

[25] Jones, B. E. Young SSMM, Antoniskis D. Relationship of the manifestations of tuberculosis to CD4 cell counts in patients with human immunodeficiency virus infection Am Rev Respir Dis (1993). , 148, 1292-1297.

[26] Pozniak, A. L, Mcleod, G. A, Ndlovu, D, et al. Clinical and chest radiographic features of tuberculosis associated with human immunodeficiency virus in Zimbabwe Am J Respir Crit Care Med (1995). , 152, 1558-1561.

[27] Light RW Tuberculous pleural effusions In: Light RW edPleural Diseases 3rd edn. Baltimore Williams & Wilkinson (1995). , 154-166.

[28] Levine, H, & Szanto, P. B. Cugell DW Tuberculous pleurisy: an acute illness Arch Intern Med (1968). , 122, 329-332.

[29] Mougdil, H, & Stridhar, G. Leitch AG Reactivation disease: the commonest form of tuberculous pleural effusion in Edinburgh 1980-1991 Respir Med (1994). , 88, 301-304.

[30] Epstein, D. M, Kline, L. R, & Abelda, S. M. Miller WT Tuberculous pleural effusions Chest (1987). , 91, 106-109.

[31] Ferrer, L. Pleural tuberculosis Eur Respir J (1997). , 10, 942-947.

[32] Chan, C. H, Arnold, M, Chan, C. Y, et al. Clinical and pathological features of tuberculous pleural effusion and its long term consequences Respiration (1991). , 58, 171-175.

[33] Valdes, L, & Alvarez, D. San Jose E. et al. Tuberculous pleurisy: a study of 254 patients Arch Intern Med (1998). , 158, 2017-2021.

[34] Shu, C. C, Wang, J. T, Wang, J. Y, et al. In hospital outcome of patients with culture-confirmed tuberculous pleurisy: clinical impact of pulmonary involvement BMC Infect Dis (2011). www.biomedcentral.com/

[35] Maher, G. G. Berger HW Massive pleural effusion: malignant and non-malignant cause in 46 patients. Am Rev Respir Dis (1972). , 105, 458-460.

[36] Hee, H. J, Lee, H. J, Kwon, S. Y, Ho, I. Y, et al. The prevalence of pulmonary parenchymal tuberculosis in patients with tuberculous Pleuritis Chest (2006). , 129, 1253-1258.

[37] Bittner, R. C, Gürvit, Ö, & Felix, R. Magnetic Resonance (MR) Imaging of the Chest: State of the Art Eur Respir J (1998). , 11, 1392-1404.

[38] Elboga, U, Yilmaz, M, Uyar, M, et al. The role of FDG PET-CT in differential diagnosis of pleural changes Rev Esp Med Nucl (2011). article in press

[39] Rossi GA; Balbi BManca F. Tuberculous pleural effusions: Evidence of selective pres-
      ence of PPD-specific T-lymphocytes at the site of inflammation in the early phase of
      infection Am Rev Respir Dis (1987). , 136, 575-579.

[40] Pai, M, & Riley, L. W. Colford JM jr. Interferon-γ-assays in the immunodiagnosis of
      tuberculosis: a systematic review The Lancet Inf Dis (2004). , 4, 761-776.

[41] Mazurek, G. H. LoBue PA, Daley CL et al. Comparison of a whole-blood interferon
      gamma assay with tuberculin skin testing for detecting latent mycobacterium tuber-
      culosis infection JAMA (2001). , 286, 1740-1747.

[42] Chegou, N. N, Walzl, G, Bolliger, C. T, et al. Evaluation of adapted whole-blood in-
      terferon-γ-release assays for the diagnostic of pleural tuberculosis Respiration
      (2008). , 76, 131-138.

[43] Hooper, C. Lee YCG, Maskell NA Interferon gamma release assays for the diagnosis
      of TB pleural effusion: hype or real Hope? Curr Opin Pulm Dis (2009). , 15, 358-365.

[44] Dewan, P. K, Grinsdale, J, & Kawamura, M. Low sensitivity of a whole-blood inter-
      feron-γ-assay for detection of active Tuberculosis Clin Infect Dis (2007). , 44, 69-73.

[45] Greco, S, Girardi, E, Masciangelo, R, et al. Adenosine deaminase and interferon gam-
      ma measurements for the diagnosis of tuberculous pleurisy: a meta-analysis Int. J.
      Tuberc. Lung Dis. (2003). , 7, 777-786.

[46] Sahn SA The diagnostic value of pleural fluid analysis Sem Respir Crit Care Med
      1995; 16:269-278

[47] Good JT JrRayle DA, Maulitz RM et al. The diagnostic value of pleural fluid pH
      Chest (1980). , 78, 55-59.

[48] Valdes, L, & Alvarez, D. San Jose E. et al. Value of adenosine in the diagnosis of tu-
      berculous pleural effusions in young patients in a region of high prevalence of tuber-
      culosis Thorax (1995). , 50, 600-603.

[49] Petterson, T, & Ojala, K. Weber TH Adenosine deaminase in pleural fluids: test for
      the diagnosis of tuberculous pleural effusions Acta Med Scand (1984). , 215, 299-304.

[50] Ungerer JPJ; Oosthuizen HMRetief JH Significance of adenosine deaminase activity
      and its isoenzymes in tuberculous effusions

[51] Hsu, W. H, & Chiang, C. D. Huang PL Diagnostic value of pleural adenosine deami-
      nase in tuberculous effusions of immunocompromised hosts J Formosan Med Ass
      (1993). , 92, 668-670.

[52] Liang, Q. L, Shi, H. Z, Wang, K, et al. Diagnostic accuracy of adenosine deaminase in
      tuberculous pleurisy: a meta analysis Respir Med (2008). , 102, 744-754.

[53] Heydermann, R. S, Makunike, R, Muza, T, et al. Pleural tuberculosis in Harare, Zim-
      babwe: the relationship between Human immunodeficiency virus, CD4 lymphocyte

count, granuloma formation and disseminated disease Tropical Med Internat Health (1998). , 3(1), 14-20.

[54] Barnes, T. W, Olson, E. J, Morgenthaler, T. I, et al. Low yield of microbiological studies on pleural fluid specimens Chest (2005). , 127, 916-921.

[55] Loddenkemper, R, Grosser, H, Mai, J, et al. Diagnostik der tuberkulösen Pleuraergüsse: prospektiver Vergleich laborchemischer, bakteriologischer, zytologischer und histologischer Untersuchungsergebnisse Prax Klein Pneumol (1983). , 37, 1153-1156.

[56] Maartens, G. Bateman ED Tuberculous pleural effusions: increased cukture yield with bedside inoculation of pleural fluid and poor diagnostic value of adenosine deaminase Thorax (1991). , 46, 96-99.

[57] Conde, M. B, Loivos, A. C, Rezende, V. M, et al. Yield of sputum induction in the diagnosis of pleural tuberculosis Am J Respir Crit Care Med (2003). , 167, 723-725.

[58] Valdes, L. San Jose E., Alvarez D. et al. Diagnosis of tuberculous pleurisy using the biologic parameters adenosine deaminase, lysozyme and interferon-γ Chest (1993). , 103, 458-465.

[59] Ribera, F, & Ocana, I. Martinez-Vasquez JM High level of interferon gamma in tuberculous pleural effusion Chest (1988). , 93, 308-311.

[60] Söderblom, T, Nyberg, P, Teppo, A. M, et al. Pleural fluid interferon gamma and tumor necrosis factor in tuberculous and rheumatoid pleurisy Eur Respir J (1996). , 9, 1652-1655.

[61] Jiang, J, Shi, H. Z, Liang, Q. L, et al. Diagnostic value of interferon-γ in tuberculous pleurisy: a metaanalysis Chest (2007). , 131, 1133-1141.

[62] Brisson-noel, A, Gicquel, B, Lecossier, D, et al. Rapid diagnosis of tuberculosis by amplification of mycobacterial DNA in clinical samples Lancet (1989). , 4, 1069-1071.

[63] Roth, A, Schaberg, T, & Mauch, H. Molecular diagnosis of tuberculosis: current clinical validity and future perspectives Eur Respir J (1997). , 10, 1877-1891.

[64] Lassence, A, Lecossier, D, Pierre, C, et al. Detection of mycobacterial DANN in pleural fluid from patients with tuberculous pleurisy by means of the polymerase chain reaction: comparison of protocols Thorax (1992). , 47, 265-269.

[65] De Wit, D, Maartens, G, & Steyn, L. A comparative study of the polymerase chain reaction and conventional prcedures fort the diagnosis of tuberculous pleural effusion Tuber Lung Dis (1992). , 73, 262-267.

[66] Querol, J. M, & Minguez, J. Garcia Sanchez E. et al. Rapid diagnosis of pleural tuberculosis by polymerase chain reaction Am J Respir Crit Care Med (1995). , 152, 1977-1981.

[67]   Salian, N. V, Rish, J. A, Eisenach, K. D, & Cave, M. D. Bates JH Polymerase chain re-
       action to detect mycobacterium tuberculosis in histologic specimens Am J Respir Crit
       Care Med (1998). , 148, 1150-1155.

[68]   Marchetti, G, Gori, A, & Catozzi, L. Evaluation of PCR in detection of mycobacteri-
       um tuberculosis from formalin-fixed paraffin-embedded tissues: comparison of four
       amplification assays J Clin Microbiol (1998). , 36, 1512-1517.

[69]   Gamboa, F, Fernandez, G, Padilla, E, et al. Comparative evaluation of initial and new
       versions of the gene-probe amplified mycobacterium tuberculosis in respiratory and
       non-respiratory specimens J Clin Microiol (1998). , 36, 684-689.

[70]   Palacios, J. J, Ferro, J, Ruiz-palma, N, et al. Comparison of the ligase chain reaction
       with solid and liquid culture media for routine detection of mycobacterium tubercu-
       losis in non-respiratory specimens Eur J Clin Microbiol Infect Dis (1998). , 17,
       767-772.

[71]   Ruiz-manzano, J, Manterola, J. M, Gamboa, F, et al. Detection of mycobacterium tu-
       berculosis in paraffin-embedde pleural biopsy specimens by commercial ribosomal
       RNA and DNA amplification kits Chest (2000). , 118, 648-655.

[72]   Pai, M, Flores, L. L, Hubbard, A, et al. Nucleic Acid amplification tests in the diagno-
       sis of tuberculous pleuritis: a systematic review and meta analyses BMC Infectious
       Disease (2004). www.biomedcentral.com/

[73]   Dinnes, J, Deeks, J, Kunst, H, et al. A systematic review of rapid diagnostic tests for
       the detection of tuberculous infection Health Tecnol Assess (2007). , 11, 1-196.

[74]   Kirsch, C. M, Kroe, D. M, Azzi, T. L, et al. The optimal number of pleural biopsy
       specimens for a diagnosis of tuberculous pleurisy Chest (1997). , 112, 702-706.

[75]   Loddenkemper, R, Mai, J, & Scheffler, N. Brandt HJ Wertigkeit bioptischer Verfahren
       beim Pleuraerguss: Individueller Vergleich zwischen Exsudatuntersuchung, Stanz-
       biopsie und Thorakoskopie Prax Klin Pneumol (1978). , 32, 334-343.

[76]   Diacon, A. H, & Van De, B. W. Wal, C. Wyser, JP Smedema, J. Bezuidenhout, CT Bol-
       liger, G. Walzl Diagnostic tools in tuberculous pleurisy: a direct comparative study
       Eur Respir J (2003). , 22, 589-591.

[77]   Colt HG Thoracoscopy: window to the pleural space Chest 1999; 107:1409-1415

[78]   Jocabaeus HC Über die Möglichkeit die Zystoskopie bei der Untersuchung seröser
       Höhlen anzuwenden Münch Med Wschr [1910] 40:2090-2092

[79]   Loddenkemper R Thoracoscopy: state of the Art Eur Respir J 1998; 11:213-221

[80]   Mathur, P. N, Boutin, C, & Loddenkemper, R. Medical thoracoscopy: techniques and
       indications in pulmonary medicine J Bronchiol (1994). , 1, 1153-1156.

[81] Harris, R. J, & Kavuru, M. S. Mehta ACThe impact of thoracoscopy on the management of pleural disease Chest (1996). , 107, 845-852.

[82] Blumberg, H. M, Burman, W. J, Chaisson, R. E, et al. American Thoracic Society/ Centers for Disease Control and Prevention / Infectious Disease Society of America: treatment of tuberculosis Am J Respir Crit Care Med (2003). , 167, 603-662.

[83] Lee, C. H, & Wang, C. J. Lan RS Corticosteroids in the treatment of tuberculous pleurisy: a double-blind, placebo-controlled, randomised study Chest (1988). , 94, 1256-1259.

[84] Wyser, C, & Walzl, G. Smedema JP Corticosteroids in the treatment of tuberculous pleurisy: a double-blind, placebo-controlled, randomised study. Chest (1996). , 110, 333-338.

[85] Galarza, I, Canete, C, & Granados, A. Randomised trial of corticosteroids in the treatment of tuberculous pleurisy Thorax (1999). , 50, 1305-1307.

[86] Chung, C. L, Chen, C. L, Yeh, C. Y, et al. Early effective drainage in the treatment of loculated tuberculous pleurisy Eur Respir J (2008). , 31, 1261-1267.

[87] Pablo de AVillena V., Echave-Sustaeta L., Encuentra AL Are pleural fluid parameters related to the development of residual pleural thickening in tuberculosis? Chest (1997). , 112, 1293-1297.

[88] Iuchi K, Aozasa K, Yamamoto S et al. Non-Hodgkin's lymphoma of the pleural cavity developing from longstanding pyothorax. Summary of clinical and pathological findings in thirty-seven cases Jpn J Clin Oncol (1989) 19(3):249-57

Miscellaneous

Chapter 3

Peadiatric Tuberculosis: Is the World Doing Enough?

Claude Kirimuhuzya

Additional information is available at the end of the chapter

1. Introduction

Until recently, tuberculosis (TB) had become a neglected disease, particularly in children. It was after the emergence of multi drug resistant TB, and the complications brought about by the HIV/AIDS coinfection, that TB took centre stage again. The common perception has been that children rarely develop severe forms of TB and that they do not contribute much to the spread of the epidemic. Although this could be the case in non-endemic areas, where diligent contact tracing is enforced, in children from endemic areas it is a different story as revealed by an autopsy study conducted in Zambia which demonstrated that tuberculosis was a major cause of death from respiratory disease (Chintu et al., 2002).

Children are particularly vulnerable to more rapid development of severe disease and death after infection, and those with latent infection become the reservoir of disease reactivation in adulthood, fueling the future epidemic (Nicol et al., 2011). Since focus has been on reducing transmission, previous TB control strategies have not prioritized childhood TB (Zar and Pai, 2011). Due to the difficulty in establishing an accurate diagnosis of childhood tuberculosis, the true extent of the tuberculosis-related morbidity and mortality suffered by children in endemic areas is rarely appreciated (Chintu et al., 2002). For example, Regional Data from the WHO in 2007 showed that smear-positive TB in children aged under 14 years accounted for 0.6–3.6% of reported cases but since about 95% of cases in children under 12 years of age are smear negative, these data underestimate the true burden of TB. Furthermore, in countries with a high prevalence of HIV infection, there has been a marked increase in the incidence and a decrease in the peak age prevalence of infectious TB; thus, most cases now occur in young adults, who are often parents of young children (WHO Report, 2009). This finding suggests that children in developing countries will emerge as a group at high risk. In industrialized countries, most childhood TB cases are detected through contact tracing and have good outcomes. This is in contrast to the situation in low- and middle-income countries, where childhood TB is closely associated with poverty, overcrowding, and malnutrition, with consequently higher death and lower treatment success rates (Nelson and Wells, 2010).

Studies have revealed that children contribute a significant proportion to the disease burden and suffer severe tuberculosis-related morbidity and mortality, particularly in endemic areas. TB is now among the 10 major causes of mortality among children, with a global estimate of 130,000 deaths per year (WHO Report, 2009). Mortality has a strong correlation with socioeconomic status, underlying nutritional status and immunocompetence (Palme, 2002). TB has also been reported to be the third most common cause of death in HIV-infected children with a clinical diagnosis of acute severe pneumonia (Palme, 2002). With roughly a million cases estimated globally each year (Walls and, Shingadia, 2004) and a much higher risk of severe disease and death among young children than adults, paediatric TB remains a public health emergency and this is particularly evident in developing countries with poor public health infrastructure.

As in adults, the majority of cases occur in the 22 high burden countries, where a combination of high transmission rates and a large proportion of the population under the age of 15 years mean children account for up to 25-40% of cases, with incidence rates for paediatric TB ranging from 60-600 per 100,000 per year (Nelson and Wells, 2004). Increasing rates of childhood TB have also been reported in Eastern Europe in the wake of the explosive TB epidemic which followed the break up of the Soviet Union (Walls and Shingadia, 2007). Even traditionally low-burden countries have seen a rise in cases, mainly due to immigration from TB endemic areas. In most countries of Western Europe and North America, where children account for 4-7% cases, paediatric incidence rates vary from about 1 to 15 per 100,000 per year, although much higher rates are observed in some cities, such as London (Newton et al., 2008).

Despite this huge disease burden, children's access to anti-tuberculosis treatment in most endemic areas remains poor, as tuberculosis control programs focus predominantly on the treatment of sputum smear–positive adults (Starke, 2002). Recent technological advancements in diagnosis of TB in adults have not been validated in children and, similarly, trials of new drugs and development of pediatric formulations of standard first- and second-line drugs are lagging behind. As a result both research and surveillance data in the field of childhood TB have been greatly limited. Further research into the epidemiology, immune mechanisms, diagnosis, treatment and prevention of childhood TB is urgently needed to enhance our understanding of TB in children which may provide wider insights and opportunities to facilitate efforts to control TB in the population.

Another problem is that most programs for TB control are limited because they target and treat only active cases (Graham, et al., 2004) when most TB cases in children present as latent tuberculosis infection (LTBI) with active disease occurring mainly in developing countries (Dogra, et al., 2007). Without treatment, the majority of infants aged under 1 year die due to TB. Even with effective antimicrobial therapy, severe TB continues to occur in young children (Ávalos and Montes de Oca, 2012). Priorities for future research should, therefore, enhance collaborations between developing and developed nations.

This chapter addresses some of the unique features of TB in children; presents existing and novel diagnostic, therapeutic and preventative measures; and outlines important areas of future research. The main challenges for future research are highlighted and in conclusion it is emphasized that well-targeted interventions, improved resources, and improved political commitment, may lead to a dramatic reduction in tuberculosis-related morbidity and mortality among children.

2. Epidemiology of paediatric TB

2.1. Global disease burden of paediatric TB

Poor case ascertainment, lack of resources for active case finding in most settings, and limited paediatric surveillance data from TB control programs all hamper efforts to define accurately the global burden of childhood TB (Nelson and Wells, 2004). Until recently, under the WHO Directly Observed Treatment Short Course (DOTS) strategy, only smear positive cases were being reported for children, yet smears are seldom performed in many high burden settings and most disease in children is smear negative.

Although limited surveillance data prevent reliable estimates of the contribution of TB to childhood mortality, available data indicate that pneumonia is the commonest cause of childhood death globally (Nelson et al., 2004) an implication that TB, being an important cause of pneumonia in many settings (Scott et al., 2008), may contribute significantly to these global childhood deaths. A necropsy study in Zambia found evidence of TB in 18% of HIV-positive and 26% of HIV-negative children dying of pneumonia (Chintu et al., 2002) although more robust regional data on the epidemiology of childhood TB are urgently needed to define the true burden of disease, and to characterize current transmission rates and circulating strains.

2.2. Pathophysiology of TB in children

2.2.1. Natural history of TB in children

The natural history of TB in children and pediatric patients follows a series of steps in which phase 1 occurs after an incubation period of 3–8 weeks after primary infection. This is followed by appearance of well-defined signs that include fever, erythema nodosum, a positive tuberculin skin test response, and formation of the primary complex visible on chest radiography. Phase 2 occurs 1–3 months after the phase 1 in which period, the bacillus can migrate to other parts of the body via the blood and this represents the period of the highest risk for the development of tuberculous meningitis and miliary tuberculosis in young children. This is the phase where dissemination of the bacillus most frequently occurs. Phase 3 occurs 3–7 months after primary infection and is the period of pleural effusions in children greater than 5 years old and bronchial disease in children less than 5 years. Phase 4 presents after 1–3 years after phase 1 and is during which the osteoarticular tuberculosis in children 5 years and below, appears. Phase 5 occurs up to 3 years after phase 1 and it is presented after calcification has been completed. It is after this stage that manifestations of classical adult tuberculosis appear (Marais et al., 2004).

Extrapulmonary tuberculosis or miliary TB is a complication of primary TB in young children. It includes peripheral lymphadenopathy, TB meningitis, skeletal TB, and other organ involvement. Other unusual sites for TB include the middle ear, gastrointestinal (GI) tract, skin, kidneys, and ocular structures (Marais et al., 2006). Lymph node involvement typically occurs 6-9 months following initial infection by the tubercle bacilli. More superficial lymph nodes commonly are involved. Frequent sites of involvement include the anterior cervical, submandibular, and supraclavicular nodes. TB of the skeletal system may lead to involvement of the inguinal, epitrochlear, or axillary lymph nodes. Typically, infected lymph nodes are firm and non- tender with non erythematous overlying skin. The nodes are initially non-fluctuant. Suppuration and spontaneous drainage of the lymph nodes may occur with caseation and the development of necrosis (Marais et al., 2006).

Bone or joint TB or skeletal TB may present acutely or sub-acutely. Vertebral disease may go unrecognized for months to years because of its indolent nature. Common sites involved include the large weight-bearing bones or joints, including the vertebrae (50%), hip (15%), and knee (15%). Destruction of the bones with deformity is a late sign of TB. Manifestations for skeletal TB may include angulation of the spine (gibbus deformity) and/or Pott disease (severe kyphosis with destruction of the vertebral bodies). Cervical spine involvement may result in allantoaxial subluxation, which may lead to paraplegia or quadriplegia.

2.2.2. TB risk factors

Following infection children have a higher risk not only of progression to disease, but also of extrapulmonary dissemination and death. Infants have a particularly high morbidity and mortality from TB (WHO, 2007). While many factors including host genetics, microbial virulence and underlying conditions that impair immune competence (as is the case with malnutrition and HIV infection) determine the outcome of infection, it is likely that the high rate of progressive TB seen in young children is largely a reflection of the immaturity of the immune response. Risk factors for the acquisition of tuberculosis (TB) are usually exogenous to the patient. Thus, the likelihood of being infected depends on the environment and the features of the index case. However, the development of TB disease depends on inherent immunologic status of the host. For example, tuberculosis has been reported in patients treated for arthritis, inflammatory bowel disease, and other conditions with tumor necrosis factor (TNF)-alpha blockers/antagonists.

2.2.3. Factors for acquiring paediatric TB disease

Neonatal CD4 cells appear intrinsically deficient in their capacity to express Th1 effector function, partially attributed to hypermethylation of the proximal promoter of the IFN-γ gene, (White et al., 2002) and this results in a highly restricted pattern of IFN-γ response to a variety of stimuli (Kampmann et al., 2006). CD154 (CD40 ligand) expression is also significantly reduced compared with adult cells. These findings of generally impaired cell-mediated immune responses in the neonate and young children raise the question of whether antigen-specific immune responses to mycobacteria are equally affected. Delayed type hypersensitivity (DTH) to purified protein derivative (PPD) may be absent in up to 40% of HIV negative children presenting with extrapulmonary TB, (van der Weert et al., 2006) compounding the difficulties of diagnosis in young children. However, studies measuring responses to neonatal vaccination with M. bovis BCG demonstrate potent Th1 responses, possibly related to the activating properties of BCG vaccine on the potent antigen-presenting cells (APC). Indeed while the long term efficacy of BCG vaccination may be limited, it does offer protection against disseminated disease in infants and young children. The risk of serious and potentially devastating disease is nevertheless still high in the first two years of life, underscoring the need for a better understanding of the determinants of host protection particularly in this vulnerable age group.

In the natural history of childhood intrathoracic TB, primary infection before 2 years of age frequently progresses to disease within the first 12 months (Marais, et al., 2004). Young age and HIV infection are the most important risk factors for severe or disseminated disease; the risk of disease progression decreases during childhood, least at 5–10 years of age, and increases again during adolescence. Pulmonary parenchymal disease and intrathoracic adenopathy are the most common clinical manifestations of pediatric TB, accounting for 60%–80% of all cases (Jensen, 2002). Among extra-pulmonary manifestations, lymphadenopathy is the most common (67%), followed by central nervous system involvement (13%) and pleural (6%), disseminated (5%), and skeletal (4%) TB (Marais, 2006). Disseminated disease and TB meningitis are usually found in very young children (age, under 3 years) and/or HIV-infected children (Starke, 2003). More research is required to identify better strategies for case detection and contact tracing, especially in high-burden settings, and to study the role of genetic and nutritional factors that protect children from TB infection and disease.

HIV-infected children are at risk of both atypical pulmonary presentation and extra-pulmonary disease, which comprises up to 60% of TB in this population (Starke, 2003). Symptom-based diagnostic approaches perform poorly, because other HIV-related conditions, such as lymphocytic interstitial pneumonitis, broncho-ectasis, and respiratory infections (including viral pneumonitis), mimic the clinical and radiographic features of TB (Marais, 2007). Lymphocytic interstitial pneumonitis tends to occur in children aged less than two years, presents with recurrent respiratory symptoms, and is associated with clubbing and generalized lymphadenopathy and a miliary TB-like picture on chest radiograph. Although these patients improve temporarily with antibiotic therapy, antiretroviral treatment is required for sustained benefit and to avoid development of chronic lung disease. In the short term, there is little prospect of achieving a widely available gold standard diagnosis of TB in children either by means of culture, microscopy, PCR, or serological testing. Consequently, clinicians must rely on clinical criteria, chest radiography, and tuberculin testing, and attempts must be made to improve the predictive power of available tools (Swaminathan and Rekha, 2010).

The immunological responses to MTB are due to the interaction between the immature immune system in children, the host, bacterial and environmental factors (Meya and McAdam, 2007). Genetic as well as acquired defects in host immune response pathways greatly increase the risk of progressive disease (Kampmann et al., 2005). Results from genome wide linkage studies suggest that TB disease susceptibility is highly likely to be polygenic, with contributions from many minor loci (Hill, 2006) and a large number of TB susceptibility markers have been identified from candidate gene studies as 'disease-causing' genes which include TIRAP, HLA DQB1, VDR, IL-12β, IL12Rβ1, IFN-γ, SLC11A1 and MCP-1. However, to date the greatest evidence to support an underlying genetic basis for TB has come from the discovery of single gene defects predisposing to disseminated and often lethal mycobacterial disease. Most observations were initially made in children with reduced ability to activate macrophage antimycobacterial mechanisms through defects in the IFN-γ (Kampmann et al., 2005) /IL-12 pathway resulting in severe mycobacterial infection. However, subsequent studies have led to description of mutations in five susceptibility genes (Ottenhoff et al., 2005) confirming that up-regulation of the macrophage through the IL-12/23-IFN-γ pathway is a fundamental step in the containment of infection with mycobacteria. However, despite a growing adult literature on the role of candidate genes from this pathway, data from children is scarce. This is surprising given the marked differences in TB pathophysiology in children, which may also reflect differences in genetic factors. Further studies of TB genetics in well-defined paediatric populations are therefore needed.

2.3. Impact of HIV epidemic paeditric TB

Studies demonstrating a higher risk of TB among HIV- children (Jeena et al., 2002) highlight the essential role of cell mediated immunity (CMI) in preventing mycobacterial dissemination (Tena et al., 2003). Poor CMI in HIV co-infection often results in disseminated disease, especially in advanced stages of HIV-infection, resulting in poorer survival compared to HIV-negative children (Palme et al., 2002). Risk of active TB in HIV co-infected children is related to both CD4 count and more indirectly also to viral load (Elenga et al., 2005).Conversely, restoration of cellular immunity with anti-retroviral therapy partially reverses TB susceptibility (Kampmann et al., 2006).

The impact of the Human Immunodeficiency Virus (HIV) epidemic on the burden of childhood TB has been less well characterized than for adults (Corbett et al., 2003). However, the observed shift in disease burden to younger adults it has caused, suggests that children are at particularly high risk of exposure as well as disease (Graham et al, 2001). Reported prevalence of HIV co-infection among children with TB range from below 5%, in industrialized settings, to over 50% in some high burden African settings (Nelson and Wells, 2004). However, it is often difficult to draw reliable inferences about the effect of HIV on TB incidence or risk from these observational data due to ascertainment bias or diagnostic bias; incomplete ascertainment of HIV status and because denominator population data on the proportion of all children infected with HIV are usually lacking. (For example, children with HIV are more likely to be investigated for TB and diagnosis is unreliable because it is affected by HIV status). Nevertheless an increased TB incidence and poorer outcome have been observed among HIV infected children in a variety of settings (Palme et al., 2002) including an estimated 20-fold increased TB incidence associated with HIV infection in a study from South Africa. Methodological constraints in some studies may explain why this has not been a universal finding (Marais et al., 2007).

2.4. Nutrition and paediatric TB

Several observational studies from adults and children show an association between mal-nutrition and TB, (Cegielski and McMurray, 2004) although proving the direction of a causal link is challenging, as TB in itself causes wasting. Diagnosis is further complicated by frequently false negative TST in malnutrition, reverting to positivity only once nutri-tion has improved. Nevertheless these observational data, coupled with experimental ani-mal data and impaired CMI observed in malnutrition, support its role as a risk factor for childhood TB (Cegielski and McMurray, 2004). However the effect of differing types and degrees of malnutrition, and the population at risk due to malnutrition in communities where both are endemic, are yet to be defined.

Among micronutrients, vitamin D deficiency has been most extensively studied, and shown to be associated with TB in UK immigrants. Its active metabolite 1-alpha, 25-dihydroxy-vitamin D modulates the host response to TB infection in numerous ways, including the induction of antimicrobial peptides such as Cathelicidin LL-37 (Martineau et al., 2007).

2.5. Host-pathogen interactions in paediatric TB

The relationship between MTB strain genotype and clinical manifestation of disease is poorly documented in children. A study in the Western Cape Province of South Africa demonstrated that the Beijing and Haarlem genotype families are significantly associated with drug resistant TB in children (Marais et al., 2006). The high prevalence of Beijing and Latin American Mediterranean (LAM) strains in children reflects considerable transmission of these genotype families in this setting (Marais et al., 2006).

Genetic markers of virulence and transmissibility, (Lopez et al., 2003) and the ability to modulate host cellular immunity have been described for the Beijing strain, HN878 (Reed, et al., 2004). Similarly the East African-Indian lineage is characterized by an LSP (Large Sequence Polymorphism) conferring an immune subverting phenotype that contributes to its persistence and outbreak potential of this lineage (Newton et al., 2006). Strain differences in immunoge-nicity may result in reduced detection by TST (Anderson et al., 2006) as documented in a London school contact tracing investigation - an extremely worrying phenomenon which may lead to underestimates of the true global burden of TB and underscores the need for new diagnostics. Most studies of strain-specific responses are derived from adult TB cases, and it remains to be established whether results are equally applicable to children. Further research to characterize strain differences in pathogenicity and induction of immune responses should include children as well as adults.

2.6. Clinical spectrum of paediatric TB disease

The clinical spectrum of childhood TB also reflects differences in the balance between the pathogen and the host immune response, with more severe disease resulting from either poor or 'over-exuberant' attempts to contain the disease. Many cases of primary TB infection in children are asymptomatic, self-healing and remain completely unnoticed or accidentally discovered at a later stage (Marais et al., 2004). In previously healthy children, what determines the differences in the host/pathogen interactions that lead to successful containment as opposed to progressive disease remains largely unknown. However, age and immunodeficiency are important factors. Thus, while an exuberant immune response, in immunocompetent adolescents, tends to result in adult-type, cavitating disease, (Marais et al., 2005) in young children and/or HIV co-infection, poor CMI is thought to allow unrestrained proliferation of bacilli with progressive parenchymal lung damage (with or without cavity formation) dissemination (Marais et al., 2005)

While dissemination can occur to almost any site, TB meningitis (TBM) is one of the commonest consequences of extra-pulmonary TB and develops three to six months after primary infection (Donald and Schoeman, 2004). It is also the most severe and potentially devastating form of childhood TB with mortality or significant long term neurological sequelae occurring in almost 50% of cases (Thwaites and Tran, 2005). Anatomical differences in children, compared with adults, also modify the presentation of TB. Complications arising from enlarging lymph nodes and small airways are common in children less than five years of age (Marais, et al., 2004; Marais et al., 2005). Post-primary TB can result in upper-lobe pulmonary consolidation and cavitation with highly infectious patients, more likely to be seen in older children.

HIV infection often mimics TB associated signs and symptoms, such as weight loss, failure to thrive and chronic pulmonary symptoms, corroborating the diagnostic difficulties (reviewed in references (Marais et al., 2007). In turn, the treatment of HIV with ART can result in unmasking signs and symptoms of underlying LTBI or active TB in the form of immune reconstitution disease (IRD) (Walters et al., 2006) in young children is largely a reflection on the immaturity of the immune response.

2.7. Differences in childhood immune responses to TB

The alveolar macrophage is the first line of defense in the innate immune response to TB and plays a critical role in amplifying the response to infection. Studies in the animal and human host have consistently demonstrated reduced microbial killing and diminished monocyte recruitment to the site of infection in infants compared to adults. Thus impairment of innate pulmonary defenses in the neonate and infant may allow mycobacteria to overwhelm the effects of the innate immune system prior to the initiation of an antigen-specific immune response.

Antigen presentation by dendritic cells (DC), the major antigen-presenting cell (APC) in the lung, and the efficiency with which naïve T cells respond to antigen, also appears less effective in infants and may contribute to the delay in initiating an appropriate antigen-specific response, resulting in development of active disease. Blood derived DCs are functionally immature at birth relative to adult DCs and continue to express a less differentiated phenotype throughout early childhood (Upham et al., 2006). Some studies also suggest that neonatal APCs lack the capacity to deliver important Th1 polarising signals to T-cells. Their capacity to synthesise interleukin (IL)-12, a key APC-derived cytokine, matures slowly during childhood (Upham et al., 2002) and neonatal, monocyte-derived DCs have a specific defect in IL-12p35 expression (Goriely et al., 2001). IL-12 is critical for the initial phases of Th1 polarisation and also for maintaining the efficiency of the interferon (IFN)-γ transcription machinery in Th1 effector cells (Goriely et al., 2001).

2.8. Latent tuberculosis in children

2.8.1. Detection of the infection

Transmission within a community is measured by the Annual Risk of Infection (ARI) (Rieder, 2005). Infection rates rise with increased exposure in toddlers, around the ages of school entry and with increased social mobility in late teens and early adulthood (Marais et al., 2004). ARI is traditionally estimated using childhood tuberculin surveys, although this has limitations due to the poor specificity of the tuberculin skin test (TST), particularly where Bacille Calmette Guerin (BCG) vaccine is given at birth and non-tuberculous mycobacteria (NTM) are endemic. T-cell based interferon gamma release assays (IGRAs) may offer a more specific alternative (Dinnes et al., 2007), but have not yet found a use in this context due to their cost, ethical concerns about venepuncture in healthy children (Rieder, 2005), and uncertainty about the significance of a positive result for later development of active disease. Threfore, differences in the pathophysiology and clinical presentation of TB in children make diagnosis more challenging than in adults (Shingadia and Novelli, 2003) and the definitions of latent infection and disease, are less clear cut (Marais et al., 2004).

2.8.2. Activation from infection to disease

Following infection, several factors appear to influence the balance of risk between latent TB infection (LTBI) or progression to active disease, including age (Marais et al., 2004) and nutritional (Cegielski and McMurray, 2004), vaccination and immune status (Chen, 2004). Children are at much higher risk of progression to active disease than adults. This risk is greatest for infants and children under 2 years of age (Marais et al., 2004). Active surveillance data from the pre-chemotherapy era suggest that the majority of children develop radiological abnormalities following infection, including 60-80% of children less than two years. However, less than 10% of those are notified, suggesting the disease is controlled by the host immune response in most cases (Marais et al., 2004). This has implications for case definitions based on radiological findings. Overall the risk of disease is highest among infants and in late teens, with the lowest risk between 5 and 10 years - the so-called "safe school years" (Marais et al., 2004). Most disease occurred in the first year following infection (Marais et al., 2004). Thus because disease in young children reflects recent infection, rather than secondary reactivation, the paediatric disease burden potentially provides a useful measure of current transmission

within a community, Marais et al., 2005) including multi-drug resistant (MDR) (Schaaf et al., 2006) and extensively drug resistant (XDR) strains.

3. Challenges presented by paediatric TB in the field of diagnosis and treatment

3.1. Concepts from the natural history of disease

The pre-chemotherapy literature documented the natural history of tuberculosis in children. Unfortunately, clinicians and researchers have limited access to these important studies as they were conducted before 1950 and are not included in modern electronic databanks. Since the discovery of safe and effective antituberculosis treatment, conducting studies on the natural history of disease became unethical and therefore these historic disease descriptions remain invaluable today. The pre-chemotherapy literature provides a strong body of evidence; multiple studies monitored large cohorts of children for prolonged periods of time and carefully documented the development of disease after primary infection with Mycobacterium tuberculosis. A critical review of the natural history of disease identified three central concepts that are important to consider when addressing current and/or future challenges in the field of childhood tuberculosis: (1) the need for accurate case definitions, (2) the importance of risk stratification, and (3) the diverse spectrum of disease pathology, which necessitates accurate disease classification (Marais et al., 2004).

3.2. Challenge of case definition

Accurate case definition revolves mainly around the ability to differentiate primary infection from active disease. Primary infection is believed to occur when a previously uninfected child inhales a single infectious aerosol droplet, which may contain fewer than five bacilli that penetrate into a terminal airway. A localized pneumonic process, referred to as the primary parenchymal (Ghon) focus, results at the site of organism deposition. For the first 4–6 weeks, unrestrained multiplication occurs within the Ghon focus and bacilli drain via local lymphatics to the regional lymph nodes and beyond. The upper lobes drain to ipsilateral–paratracheal nodes, whereas the rest of the lung drains to perihilar and subcarinal nodes, with dominant lymph flow from left to right (Marais et al., 2006). The Ghon complex is represented by both the Ghon focus, with or without some overlying pleural reaction, and the affected regional lymph nodes (Marais et al., 2006).

Occult dissemination frequently occurs during this early proliferative phase before cell-mediated immunity is fully activated. Bacteriologic cultures collected at this time may be positive; Wallgren demonstrated in the 1930s that M. tuberculosis is sometimes recovered from recently infected children who are not diseased. Therefore, with active contact tracing and aggressive screening that includes the collection of mycobacterial cultures in asymptomatic children it is not unexpected to find some positive cultures in recently infected children who are not diseased. This illustrates the overlap that exists between recent primary infection and case definitions of disease that rely exclusively on bacteriology. It is important to consider this overlap when case definitions are formulated for research purposes, particularly within the contact setting, although it is less relevant in everyday practice where there is no reason to obtain cultures from completely asymptomatic children.

Uncomplicated hilar adenopathy remains the most common disease manifestation in children and is usually regarded as the hallmark of primary tuberculosis. However, the prechemotherapy literature documented transient hilar adenopathy in the majority (50–60%) of children after recent primary pulmonary infection, of whom only a few progressed to disease (Marais et al., 2004). The natural history of disease illustrates that progression to disease is indicated by the onset of persistent, nonremitting symptoms, referred to as the breakpoint of clinical significance whereas the complete absence of symptoms usually indicates good organism containment (Marais et al., 2004). By convention, asymptomatic hilar adenopathy is currently treated as active disease, although early experience with isoniazid alone demonstrated that one-drug therapy was sufficient in these cases. In terms of pathophysiology, microbiology, and natural history, asymptomatic hilar adenopathy is more indicative of recent primary infection than active disease (Marais et al., 2004).

This indicates that radiologic signs should be interpreted with caution in the absence of clinical data. The entity of so-called asymptomatic tuberculosis, where the case definition rests exclusively on radiographic criteria, is a case in point. High-resolution computed tomography is the most sensitive tool available to detect hilar adenopathy (Andronikou et al., 2004), as demonstrated by the fact that in children with recent M. tuberculosis infection and a normal chest radiograph, prominent intrathoracic nodes are frequently demonstrated by high-resolution computed tomography. Particular caution is required when interpreting the relevance of these radiologic signs in the absence of clinical data. It is important to point out that there is no role for high-resolution computed tomography in the evaluation of asymptomatic, immune-competent children exposed to M. tuberculosis.

In reality, differences in patient selection may result in the use of different functional case definitions even though the definitions appear similar on paper. In non-endemic areas where active contact tracing is diligently enforced, more children with transient radiologic signs indicative of recent primary infection will be identified, and those with active disease will be diagnosed at an earlier, less advanced stage. Active contact tracing is rarely enforced in endemic areas and children usually present to health care facilities with suspicious symptoms and more advanced disease (Marais et al., 2006). Unlike asymptomatic contacts in which visible radiologic signs probably indicate recent primary infection only, radiologic signs in symptomatic children indicate active disease. From a research perspective it is important to be aware of these differences, as inconsistent case definitions may confound the scientific interpretation of results. In everyday practice, distinguishing between the signs and symptoms of recent primary infection and active disease is less relevant in high-risk children (less than 3 years of age and/or immune compromised) in whom infection frequently progresses to disease, sometimes with rapid disease progression.

3.3. Problems of risk stratification

The natural history of disease demonstrates that age is the most important variable that determines the risk to progress to disease after primary M. tuberculosis infection in immune-competent children (Marais et al., 2004). Infants are at the highest risk (Marais et al., 2004) and the risk drops but stays appreciable in the second year of life, to reach its lowest level in children infected between 5 and 10 years of age (Marais et al., 2004). Children with human immuno-deficiency virus (HIV) infection and/or other forms of immune compromise, such as severe malnutrition, seem to experience a similar high risk as the very young (less than 2 years of age), immune-immature children (Marais et al., 2004). The vast majority (more than 95%) of children who progress to disease do so within 12 months of primary infection and, therefore, it seems prudent to categorize all children less than 3 years of age and/or immune-compro-mised children as high-risk. Because of the frequency and rapidity with which disease progression may occur, exposure to and/or infection with M. tuberculosis warrants treatment intervention in this high-risk group (Marais et al., 2004).

Immune-competent children of at least 3 years of age are at low risk of progression to disease after primary infection. However, as the vast majority of children in endemic areas become infected after 2 to 3 years of age, these low-risk children still contribute a significant percentage to the total disease burden. In addition, although these children are at low risk to progress to disease, latent infection with M. tuberculosis does pose the risk of future reactivation of the disease. In non-endemic areas, where transmission rates are low and eradicating the pool of latent infection is an achievable aim, the provision of preventive therapy to these low-risk children is warranted. In endemic areas, where the majority of disease in immune-competent adults results from ongoing transmission and not from reactivation (Saiman et al., 2001), the provision of preventive therapy after exposure and/or infection becomes less relevant. The major diagnostic challenge in this low-risk group is the differentiation between latent infection and active disease (Marais et al., 2004). Fortunately, active disease is accompanied by persis-tent, non-remitting symptoms and disease progression is slow, which provides a window of opportunity for symptom-based diagnosis (Marais et al., 2004).

3.4. Difficulties in classifying disease diversity

Childhood tuberculosis is often reported as a single disease entity, although it represents a diverse spectrum of pathology (Marais et al., 2004), and one of the obstacles has been the lack of standard descriptive terminology. Accurate disease classification is important, because of its prognostic significance and to facilitate scientific communication and optimal case man-agement. Within the Ghon focus, containment is usually successful, but disease progression may result from either poor or "excessive" containment. Poor containment and unrestrained organism proliferation may cause progressive parenchymal damage, with ultimate break-down of the Ghon focus. Infants (Dinnes et al., 2007) and HIV-positive children (Pai et al., 2004), who have poor cell-mediated immune responses, are most vulnerable to this type of cavitation. In contrast, immune-competent adolescents seem to mount an "excessive" (dam-aging) immune response in an attempt to contain the organism. The exact immune mechanisms underlying adult-type disease remain uncertain, but it is a striking observation that it emerges only as children enter into puberty (Marais et al., 2004). It is important to remember that children with adult-type disease are frequently sputum smear–positive and that they do contribute to disease transmission (Cegielski and McMurray, 2004), particularly in congregate settings such as schools.

Complications that arise from affected lymph nodes are most common in children less than 5 years old, because of exuberant lymph node enlargement and small airway size (Marais et al., 2004). Extraluminal compression results when the airway is encircled by enlarged lymph nodes and associated inflammatory edema (Marais et al., 2004). Intraluminal obstruction results from polyps or granulomatous tissue that develops secondary to inflammatory changes in the bronchial wall, or when caseous material is deposited into an airway after lymph node eruption (Marais et al., 2004). Radiologic signs vary from segmental or lobar hyperinflation with partial obstruction and a check-valve effect (Marais et al., 2004), to segmental or lobar collapse with total obstruction and resorption of distal air (Marais et al., 2004). The pathology that results from the aspiration of caseous material is influenced by the dose and virulence of the bacilli aspirated. The pathology may range from transient parenchymal consolidation, resulting from a pure hypersensitivity response to dead bacilli and/or toxic products, to an expansile pneumonic process with progressive caseating pneumonia in the affected segment or lobe (Marais et al., 2004). Expansile caseating pneumonia frequently leads to parenchymal destruction and cavity formation.

Thus, cavitary disease in children may result from three distinct pathologic processes: (1) poor containment at the site of organism deposition (very young and/or immune-compromised children); (2) aspiration of live bacilli when a diseased lymph node erupts into an airway, with destructive caseating pneumonia in the distal segment or lobe (children less than 5 year of age); and (3) adult-type disease (mainly children greater than 10 year of age). The fact that immune-competent children 5 to 10 yr of age experience the lowest risk to progress to disease after primary infection with M. tuberculosis is an interesting immunologic phenomenon that is poorly understood. A better understanding of age-related differences in the immune response to M. tuberculosis may provide important insight into immune correlates of disease and protection.

Disseminated disease occurs predominantly in very young (immune-immature) and/or immune-compromised children, such as the HIV-infected or severely malnourished (Pai et al., 2004; Shingadia and Chen, 2004). These children have suboptimal cellular immune responses and demonstrate poor containment of the organism, both within the regional lymph nodes and at the multiple sites of occult dissemination. TB meningitis (TBM) is the most dangerous complication of disseminated disease, occurring in 20 to 30% of cases (Chen, 2004).

3.5. Challenges in diagnosis

3.5.1. Overview of diagnostic challenges

Diagnostic difficulties pose the greatest challenge to childhood TB management (Marais and Pai, 2007). There are diagnostic complications because: (i) TB can mimic many common child-hood diseases, including pneumonia, generalized bacterial and viral infections, malnutrition, and HIV (Marais and Pai, 2007); (ii) the absence of a practical reference test or gold standard (Marais et al., 2006); (iii) of the inability of child patients to expectorate sputum (Nelson and Wells, 2004) (iv) of the nonspecific clinical presentation (Nicol. et al., 2009); (v) of the lower bacillary load in children which is often smear negative (Detjen et al., 2007) (vi) confirmation by culture of Mycobacterium tuberculosis, usingthe gold standard of diagnosis in adult TB, rarely exceeds 30–40% sensitivity (although it may be considerably higher in children with advanced disease) (Hesseling et al., 2002) even when using gastric aspirates, induced sputum, liquid media, and polymerase chain reaction (PCR) (Edwards et al., 2007); vii) distinguishing between recent primary infection and active disease is highly difficult (Gomez-Pastrana et al., 2001); viii) gastric aspirates continue to be the best specimens for testing for suspected pulmonary TB in children (Ling et al., 2011) with 30–40% sensitivity (Hesseling et al., 2002).

Bacteriologic confirmation, the accepted gold standard, is of limited use in children because of the paucibacillary nature of their disease and poor bacteriologic yields. Sputum smear microscopy, often the only diagnostic test available in endemic areas, is positive in less than 10 to 15% of children with probable tuberculosis (Schaaf et al., 2006). However, the yield is high in children with adult-type disease and sputum smear microscopy has definite diagnostic value in older children (more than 10 year of age) (Cegielski and McMurray, 2004). Culture yields are also low; reported yields in children with probable tuberculosis are less than 30 to 40% (Schaaf et al., 2006). However, the bacteriologic yield depends on the specific intrathoracic disease manifestation. A study from South Africa reported a yield of 77% in children with advanced intrathoracic disease, whereas the yield in those with uncomplicated hilar adenopathy was only 35% (odds ratio, 6.3; 95% confidence interval, 3.2–12.8) (Graham et al., 2001). This indicates the potential value of sensitive bacteriology-based diagnostic approaches, particularly in endemic areas where children frequently present with advanced disease.

Most children with TB are classified as smear-negative pulmonary TB (PTB) for the reasons mentioned above, which is an inappropriate term as a smear or culture has not usually been done. This leads to difficulties in determining the true extent of PTB in children in different areas and circumstances. Extrapulmonary TB (EPTB) accounts for up to 20–30% of the total caseload of TB in children, and the diagnosis is usually easier than PTB because of the characteristic clinical features like lymphadenopathy with or without scrofula, spinal deformity, disseminated disease, meningitis, effusions (pleural or pericardial), or painless ascite (Lewinsohn et al., 2004). The isolation of Mycobacterium tuberculosis takes several weeks. Consequently, the diagnosis of TB in children is often supported only by epidemiological, clinical, and radiographic findings in the presence of a positive tuberculin skin test (López Ávalos and Montes de Oca, 2012).

The value of the classic diagnostic is based on: (1) exposure to an adult index case; (2) chronic respiratory symptoms that do not respond to broad-spectrum antibiotics; (3) documented weight loss or failure to thrive; (4) a positive tuberculin skin test (TST); (5) the presence of suggestive signs on the chest radiograph (CXR), which is greatly reduced in endemic areas where exposure to and/or infection with M. tuberculosis is common (Marais et al., 2006). These criteria are less helpful in endemic areas where a positive TST result is common and exposure to M. tuberculosis is often undocumented (Hesseling et al., 2002). For all these reasons, many children with TB are never diagnosed or registered as cases of TB (Nelson and Wells, 2004). Furthermore, the consequences of missed diagnosis in children are severe, as untreated children have a high probability of developing active TB, usually within two years of infection (López Ávalos and Montes de Oca, 2012).

The difficulty to obtain samples for TB diagnosis in children has led researchers to create smart approaches as "la cuerda dulce" (sweet string), reported by Chow et al., (2006). They provide a technique which consists of a coiled nylon string inside a gel capsule. The string unravels through a hole in the end of the weighted capsule as it descends into the stomach and the capsule then dissolves in it, allowing the string to become coated with gastrointestinal secretions containing whatever pathogens are present. After about four hours, the capsule is passed in the feces. This methodology is well tolerated by children and is less invasive than the gastrointestinal lavage (López Ávalos and Montes de Oca, 2012).

In addition to poor bacteriologic yields, the collection of bacteriologic specimens is often problematic. Two or three fasting gastric aspirates collected on consecutive days, usually requiring hospital admission, are routinely performed in young children who cannot cough up phlegm. A retrospective study from California compared the bacteriologic yield achieved in gastric aspirates collected from hospitalized and nonhospitalized children. Although the yield in hospitalized children was higher (percentage of positive cultures, 48 compared to 37%), this difference was not statistically significant, which suggests that hospitalization may not be a prerequisite for the collection of a good gastric aspirate specimen. Bronchoalveolar lavage, using flexible fiberoptic bronchoscopy, has additive value when used in combination with gastric lavage, but this technique is highly specialized and is unavailable in most endemic areas. In a study from Peru, midmorning nasopharyngeal aspiration was compared with early morning gastric aspiration; gastric aspiration provided a slightly better yield than nasopharyngeal aspiration (38 compared to 30%), but the results were comparable (Nelson et al., 2004). Nasopharyngeal aspiration is minimally invasive, does not require hospitalization or fasting, and can be performed any time of the day. A study from South Africa demonstrated that a single specimen, using hypertonic saline–induced sputum collection, may provide the same yield as three gastric aspirate specimens (Corbett et al., 2003). However, the overall yield in this study remained poor (15% with one and 20% with three induced sputum specimens) and the technique has not been used outside the hospital setting. Additional studies are awaited to confirm the feasibility and diagnostic value of collecting induced sputum specimens in primary health care settings.

Because of the difficulty in achieving bacteriologic confirmation, the diagnosis of childhood tuberculosis in non- endemic areas is usually based on (1) known contact with an adult index case (frequently within the household), (2) a positive tuberculin skin test (TST), and (3) suggestive signs on the chest radiograph. This triad provides a fairly accurate diagnosis in settings where exposure to M. tuberculosis is rare and well documented. However, its diagnostic accuracy is greatly reduced in endemic areas where exposure to M. tuberculosis is common and often undocumented, as exposure frequently occurs outside the household. Despite reservations about the specificity of the TST response after Bacille Calmette-Guérin (BCG) vaccination and/or exposure to environmental mycobacteria, a positive TST reactio remains a fairly accurate measure of M. tuberculosis infection in immune-competent children. Current U.S. guidelines recommend the use of three different cutoff points to define a positive TST reaction. In endemic areas a positive TST is not uncommon in randomly selected healthy children (Jeena et al., 2002), which limits its diagnostic value. Consequently, the diagnosis of tuberculosis in children from endemic areas depends mainly on clinical features and the subjective interpretation of the chest radiograph (Marais et al., 2007). However, chest radiography is unavailable in many endemic areas and it has well-known limitations that may result in both under- and overdiagnosis of disease (Brent et al., 2007). Despite these limitations it provides an accurate diagnosis in the majority of symptomatic children with tuberculosis and the interpretation of the chest radiograph remains the most widely used diagnostic criterion in clinical practice (Palme et al., 2002).

Various clinical scoring systems have been developed. A critical review of these clinical scoring systems concluded that they are limited by a lack of standard symptom definitions and adequate validation (Walls and Shingadia, 2007). Developing standard symptom definitions through consensus of expert opinion is a difficult and subjective exercise; better guidance may be provided by objectively measuring the potential diagnostic value of different symptom definitions. A community-based survey demonstrated that the poorly defined symptoms traditionally associated with tuberculosis (such as a cough greater than 3 weeks in duration) are frequently reported in a random selection of healthy children (Bryce et al., 2005). Of 1,397 children without tuberculosis, 253 (26.4%) reported a cough during the preceding 3 months and 66 (6.9%) reported a cough greater than 3 weeks in duration (Bryce et al., 2005). In addition, nearly 50% of children with visible hilar adenopathy on the chest radiograph (diagnosed with tuberculosis) reported no symptoms at all (Bryce et al., 2005). These observations demonstrate the limited diagnostic value of poorly defined symptoms and the need for improved symptom and case definitions. In a follow-on study the use of well-defined symptoms with a persistent, nonremitting character showed greatly improved diagnostic accuracy (Scot et al., 2008). However, the potential diagnostic value offered by the use of these well-defined symptoms requires further validation in a prospective, community-based study that includes children from all relevant risk groups. It is expected that symptom-based diagnostic approaches would have less value in high-risk children (less than 3 years of age and/or immune compromised) where disease progression may occur rapidly, emphasizing the need for preventive chemotherapy and early diagnosis of disease in this group (Chintu, et al., 2002). Other diagnostic modalities may hold promise, but have not shown convincing results to date (WHO, 2006).

Serologic tests are currently unable to diagnose childhood tuberculosis with accuracy, and sputum-based polymerase chain reaction (PCR) tests have shown variable results and limited utility (WHO, 2007). Good results were reported with the use of a heminested PCR technique in Peru, but the study used uninfected children as the control group and therefore could not evaluate the ability of this novel PCR-based test to differentiate latent infection from active disease (Upham et al., 2006), which is important, as specific concerns have been raised regarding the specificity of PCR-based tests.

The diagnostic dilemma is even more pronounced in HIV-infected children. The specificity of symptom-based diagnostic approaches is reduced by the presence of chronic HIV-related symptoms, while the potential window for symptom-based diagnosis is limited by the rapidity with which disease progression may occur. Chest radiograph interpretation is complicated by HIV-related comorbidity and atypical disease presentation. These difficulties increase the potential diagnostic value of sensitive bacteriology-based approaches, to identify HIV-infected children with tuberculosis (Upham et al., 2002). However, as HIV-infected children are in the high-risk group the detection of M. tuberculosis infection is also highly relevant. Disease progression may occur soon (less than 12 months) after primary or reinfection, or latent infection may be reactivated at a later date because of a decline in immunity. The traditional TST has poor sensitivity to detect M. tuberculosis infection in HIV-infected children; 50% or less of HIV-infected children with bacteriologically confirmed tuberculosis are TST positive, despite using an induration size of at least 5 mm (Upham et al., 2002). This is a major limitation and development of a more reliable measure of infection will be valuable to identify HIV-infected children who may benefit from preventive chemotherapy; it may also provide supportive evidence to establish a diagnosis of active tuberculosis.

3.5.2. Challenges presented by diagnosis of latent infection in children

LTBI, in children as in adults, lacks a diagnostic gold standard. The diagnosis is usually pursued after a documented household exposure, or to evaluate if chemoprophylactic therapy is indicated in the context of immunosuppression. In this setting, pre-existing MTB specific host immune responses are measured to confirm previous infection. Data in adults have confirmed that IGRA are more sensitive and specific than the TST (Pai et al., 2004; Ferrara et al., 2006) in this context. Preliminary data suggest IGRA also perform better in children but age-related data are still sparse. Longitudinal studies assessing their positive predictive value for the development of active TB are required in both TB-endemic and low-incidence countries, as the continued exposure in TB endemic settings might yield very different results, compared to the "one-off" exposure more typically encountered in non-endemic countries.

3.6. Challenges presented by drug resistance

There were an estimated 0.5 million adult cases of MDR-TB in 2007. By the end of 2008, 55 countries and territories had reported at least 1 case of extensively drug-resistant TB (WHO Report, 2009). Latest research reports published in The Lancet at the end of August 2012, indicate that researchers have found rates of both multi drug-resistant TB (MDR-TB) and extensively drug-resistant TB (XDR-TB) higher than previously thought and that they are threatening global efforts to curb the spread of TB. They contend that most international recommendations for TB control have been developed for MDR-TB prevalence of up to around 5 percent but that now the world faces a prevalence up to 10 times higher in some places, where almost half of the patients are transmitting MDR strains. The Researchers who studied rates of the disease in Estonia, Latvia, Peru, the Philippines, Russia, South Africa, South Korea, and Thailand are reported to have found that almost 44 percent of cases of MDR TB were also resistant to at least one second-line drug outline goes here (Dalton et al., 2012)

Comprehensive studies on resistance to anti-TB drugs in children are lacking, because they are not included in global surveys. Surveillance of anti-TB drug resistance during 1995–2007 among children from South Africa showed a significant increase in resistance to INH or RIF from 6.9% to 15.1% and an increase in multidrug resistance from 2.3% to 6.7% (Schaaf et al., 2009). Drug resistance among children has been documented in clinical trials of both pulmonary and extrapulmonary TB (Rekha and Swaminathan, 2007). Management of MDR-TB is a challenge, because it requires prolonged treatment for 24 months with second-line drugs, which are more toxic and expensive than first-line drugs. According to the 2006 WHO guidelines for programmatic management of MDR-TB, an optimal regimen should include a fluoroquinolone, an injectable (capreomycin, kanamycin, or amikacin), and at least 2 of the following drugs: cycloserine, thiomides, para-amino salicylic acid, and first-line agents other than INH and RIF (WHO, 2008). Experience with second-line TB drugs in children is limited; 38 children in Peru were treated with supervised, individualized regimens consisting of 5 drugs in the national program. Despite half of these children being anemic and malnourished, treatment was well tolerated and resulted in a 95% cure rate (Drobac et al., 2006).

There is little published information on optimal treatment of latent TB infection in children in contact with patients with MDR-TB. In a 30-month follow-up of contacts of patients with MDR-TB, 5% of children who received appropriate chemoprophylaxis and 20% of those who did not receive prophylaxis developed disease (Schaaf et al., 2007). Regimens used included INH, PZA, and ethionamide or EMB. Currently, the best approach may be to perform a complete risk assessment and clinical evaluation and to individualize therapy, while keeping these children under close observation. Multicentric trials are urgently required to determine the most effective drug combinations and optimal duration of chemoprophylaxis for contacts of patients with MDR-TB.

TB is often not considered in the differential diagnosis in children, especially in low endemic settings. TB can mimic many common childhood diseases, including pneumonia, generalised bacterial and viral infections, malnutrition and HIV. However, the main impediment to the accurate diagnosis of active TB is the paucibacillary nature (containing just a few bacilli) of the disease in children. Younger children also produce smaller amounts of sputum, which is usually swallowed rather than expectorated. Bacteriological samples may be collected by conducting early morning gastric washings, a fairly unpleasant procedure that requires hospital admission and overnight-fast for up to three consecutive nights. Consequently bacteriological confirmation is the exception rather than the rule with only 10-15 % of sputum samples revealing acid fast bacilli (AFB) and culture remaining negative in around 70% of cases with probable TB (Zar et al., 2005). Without a definitive diagnosis treatment is therefore often initiated on clinical judgment, aided by algorithms based on exposure history, clinical features, chest x-ray (CXR) and TST (Marais et al., 2006). Several approaches have been taken to improve the diagnosis (Marais and Pai, 2007).

3.7. Improving bacteriological detection and rapid resistance analysis

Recent advances in bacteriological and molecular methods for the detection of MTB in patient samples aim to identify drug-resistance in parallel with detection of MTB. These include the Microscopic Observation Drug Susceptibility assay (MODS) (Moore et al., 2006), more sensitive PCR techniques (Sarmiento et al., 2003) or phage-based tests such as FASTPlaque

(Kalantri et al., 2005). This represents laudable progress, particularly in the context of increasing drug resistance. Calorimetric culture systems such as the TK medium (Kocagoz et al., 2004) and electronic-nose technology (Fend et al., 2006) are also under investigation. Among adults MODS appears to be at least as sensitive as gold standard liquid culture methods (Moore et al., 2006), Data comparing its performance in children is more limited, but MODS has been evaluated in a paediatric hospital setting and found to be more sensitive than solid media in one study (Oberhelman et al., 2006). Data validating other new methods in paediatric specimens are also lacking, yet performance may be affected by the paucibacillary nature of childhood TB. The lowest limit of detection of TB by the electronic nose for example has been reported to be 104 CFU/ml of sputum for example which is just within the range of the expected bacillary burden in paediatric specimens (Fend et al., 2006). Validation of these assays on paediatric samples is a research priority (López Ávalos G G and Montes de Oca, 2012). The introduction of GeneXpert which includes use of integrated DNA extraction and amplification systems and utilizes real-time PCR (rt-PCR) technology to both diagnose TB and detect rifampicin resistance, has given a ray of hope with paediatric TB diagnosis and rifampicin resistance (Gordetsov et al., 2008).

4. Diagnosis and treatment: Current state of affairs

4.1. Classical diagnosis

4.1.1. Clinical symptoms approach

The use of well-defined symptoms improves diagnostic accuracy of pulmonry tuberculosis (PTB) (Imaz et al., 2001). With clinical symptoms approach only, the status can be classified in two; suspected TB or probable TB. Two situations lead the clinician to suspect that a child has tuberculosis. The first is a history of chronic illness with clear symptoms: cough and/or fever, weight loss or failure to thrive, an inability to return to normal health after measles or whooping cough, fatigue, and wheezing; second, is when one or more of the following: malnutrition, lymphadenopathy, chest signs, hepatomegaly and/or splenomegaly, meningeal signs, and/or ascites is/are observed. For probable TB, in addition to suspected TB, the child presents with a positive TST, a suggestive radiological chest appearing as pleural effusion, caseation of biopsy material, poor response to 2 weeks of antibiotic treatment, and/or favourable response to antituberculous treatment (weight gain and loss of signs) (Hesseling et al., 2002).

In pediatric TB, the most common symptoms are pulmonary parenchymal disease and intrathoracic adenopathy accounting for 60–80% of all cases. Among extrapulmonary manifestations, lymphadenopathy is the most common (67%), followed by central nervous system involvement (13%), pleural (6%), miliary and/or disseminated TB (5%), and skeletal TB form (4%). Disseminated disease and TB meningitis are usually found in very young children who are below the age of 3 years, and/or HIV-infected children (Nelson et al., 2004). TB meningitis occurs when the child has contact with a suspected or confirmed case.

In general, there is a sense of skepticism regarding the potential diagnostic value of symptom-based approaches but nevertheless, the natural history of childhood tuberculosis demonstrates that symptoms may have diagnostic value if appropriate risk stratification is applied. Marais et al., (2005), evaluated whether well-defined symptoms have a diagnosis value in children and a standard symptom-based questionnaire was completed and reported symptoms were individually characterized. A tuberculin skin test (TST) and chest radiograph (CXR) were performed in all children. In this study,well-defined symptoms had excellent diagnostic value.

4.1.2. Radiologic studies

Radiography became available after the First World War, and since that time, PTB detection became easier (Marais et al., 2004). Evidence of pulmonary TB in chest radiographs varies, but usually radiographs show enlargement of hilar, mediastinal, or subcarinal lymph nodes and lung parenchymal changes with hilar lymphodenopathy with or without a focal parenchymal lesion. The most common findings are segmental hyperinflation then atelectasis, alveolar consolidation, interstitial densities, pleural effusion, and, rarely, a focal mass. Cavitation is rare in young children but is more common in adolescents, who may develop reactivation disease similar to that seen in adults (Marais. and Pai, 2007). High-resolution computed tomography is the most sensitive tool currently available to detect hilar adenopathy and/or early cavitation (Hesseling et al., 2002).

4.1.3. Diagnostic algorithms

These are point-scoring systems to make diagnostic classifications. Diagnostic algorithms were developed to deal with these diagnostic difficulties and provide the health care worker with a rational, stepwise tool to identify children in need of treatment. They are very helpful and very easy to use in countries with restricted technology, but only few of them are available especially in resource limited countries (Edwards et al., (2007). Although the natural history of tuberculosis (TB) in children follows a continuum, the American Thoracic Society (ATS) definition of stages is useful (Blumberg, et al., 2003). According to the ATS the stages are as follows:

Stage 1: Exposure has occurred, implying that the child has had recent contact with an adult who has contagious TB. The child has no physical signs or symptoms and has a negative tuberculin skin test (TST) result. Chest radiography does not reveal any changes at this stage. However, not all patients who are exposed become infected, and the TST result may not be positive for 3 months. Unfortunately, children younger than 5 years may develop disseminated TB in the form of miliary disease or TB meningitis before the TST result becomes positive. Thus, a very high index of suspicion is required when a young patient has a history of contact.

Stage 2: This second stage is heralded by a positive TST result. No signs and symptoms occur, although an incidental chest radiograph may reveal the primary complex.

Stage 3: In stage 3, TB disease occurs and is characterized by the appearance of signs and symptoms depending on the location of the disease. Radiographic abnormalities may also be seen.

Stage 4: Stage 4 is defined as TB with no current disease. This implies that the patient has a history of previous episodes of TB or abnormal, stable radiographic findings with a significant reaction to the TST and negative bacteriologic studies. No clinical findings suggesting current disease are present.

Stage 5: TB is suspected, and the diagnosis is pending. Any patient with pneumonia, pleural effusion, or a cavitary or mass lesion in the lung that does not improve with standard anti-bacterial therapy should be evaluated for tuberculosis (TB). Also, patients with fever of unknown origin, failure to thrive, significant weight loss, or unexplained lymphadenopathy should be evaluated for TB (Marais et al., 2006).

4.1.4. Mycobacterial detection and isolation

Microbiological confirmation of TB in young children is not routinely attempted in many high burden settings due to the difficulty in obtaining samples and the poor performance of smear microscopy (Nicol and Zar, 2011). Diagnosis of TB still relies primarily on examination of Acid-Fast Bacilli- (AFB-) stained smears from clinical specimens in adults, however, children with pulmonary TB usually do not cough up voluntarily, either because they do not produce sputum or because it produces discomfort. When sputum samples cannot be obtained, gastric aspirate samples are used for detection and isolation of M. Tuberculosis. Most of the current TB diagnostic methods were developed over a century ago. In 1898, Neunier became the first person to culture stomach contents for the evidence of tuberculosis in children (Marais and Pai, 2007; Lalvani and Millington, 2007), so even with this method, fewer than 20% of children with TB have a positive AFB smear of sputum or gastric aspirate.

For many years, the collection of three consecutive early morning gastric lavages or gastric aspirate samples has been the accepted method for attempting microbiological confirmation even as the yield is very low and that in many populations cannot be performed due to the lack of infrastructure. In addition low pH is known to kill tuberculous bacilli, indicating that stomach pH may inhibit TB survival for subsequent culture (Marais. and Pai, 2007). More recently, a number of less invasive alternative methods have been proposed, including induced sputum (administration of an inhaled bronchodilator followed by nebulized hypertonic 3–5% saline and then collecting nasopharyngeal aspiration or expectoration of mucus from lower respiratory tract). In the nasopharyngeal aspiration, a cannula elicits a cough reflex and the sweet string test mentioned above (Nicol and Zar, 2011). One of the methods that can be used to collect samples for microbiological analysis is the string test. This is a non-invasive collection method and is reported to be well tolerated by children as young as 4 years (Chow et al., 2006). Inducing sputum after hypertonic saline nebulization has also been shown to be feasible for young children, although the most widely used procedure is still the early-morning gastric aspiration or lavage. However, all these procedures involve hospitalization, trained personnel, and attention to infection control.

All of these alternative ways of sampling have been made to increase yield because a positive culture is regarded as the "gold standard test" to establish a definitive diagnosis of TB in a symptomatic child (Hesseling et al., 2002). If culture is negative, diagnosis is made on the basis of a positive TST. With clinical and radiographic findings suggestive of TB, and history of contact with an adult source case, the child may be diagnosed with positive TB based on symptomatology. This measure was taken because the yields in children are less than 50%. Zar et al., (2000), investigated whether sputum induction could be successfully performed in infants and young children with and without HIV and determined the utility of salbutamol-induced sputum compared to gastric lavage (GL) for the diagnosis of pulmonary tuberculosis. They concluded that sputum induction can be effectively performed and is well tolerated and safe even in infants and this induction is better than GL for the isolation of M. tuberculosis in both HIV-infected and uninfected infants and children.

Although culture on Lowenstein-Jensen medium is considered to be the gold standard, liquid culture systems (commercial and non commercial) offer the possibility of more rapid and more sensitive diagnosis of active TB and drug susceptibility but are not widely available in resource-poor settings (Brittle et al., 2009) compared mycobacterial yields and time to detection in pediatric clinical samples with use of mycobacterial growth-indicator tubes with those with use of solid Lowenstein-Jensen slants and found that the yield was substantially higher with use of mycobacterial growth-indicator tubes (11% compared to 1.6%). Furthermore, the mean time to detection could be reduced from 18.5 days to 12.4 days with use of a nutrient broth supplement; newer approaches, such as the colorimetric culture systems and phage-based tests are of interest, but limited data are available for children.

4.1.5. Smear microscopy

Advances have been done in the performance of smear microscopy for the rapid detection of MTB, for example, the concentration of specimens by centrifugation or the change of the staining of carbol fuchsin (Ziehl-Neelsen or Kinyoun) for a fluorescent dyes (auramine-rhodamine), which both increases sensitivity and reduces the time for screening (Bakir et al., 2008). However, even under optimal circumstances, the sensitivity of smear microscopy for the diagnosis of childhood TB remains less than 15%, except in older children with adult-like disease (Nicol and Zar, 2011).

4.1.6. Tuberculin skin test (TST)

This is one of the major classes of tests that are currently used to detect Latent TB. Tuberculin which is also called purified protein derivative or PPD is a standardised killed extract of cultured TB, which is injected into the skin to estimate an individual's immune response to TB. There are three methods of testing: the Mantoux test, the Heaf test and the Tine test but not all of them are currently available for use and some countries prefer one over the other. The Heaf test is no loner available because its continued manufacture was not economically viable.

The Tuberculin skin test, or Mantoux TST, is based on the detection of a cutaneous delayed-type hypersensitivity response to purified protein derivative, a poorly defined mixture of antigens present in M. tuberculosis, Mycobacterium bovis Bacille Calmette-Guerin (BCG) and several nontuberculous mycobacteria (Nicol et al., 2011). TST is the standard method for detecting infection by M. tuberculosis. The reaction is measured as millimeters of induration after 48 to 72 hours. This test was the only method available for the diagnosis of latent tuberculosis infection (LTBI) until very recently.

The Heaf test uses what is called a Heaf gun which uses disposable single-use heads, each head having six needles arranged in a circle. The device has standard heads and pediatric heads - the standard head being used on all patients aged 2 years and older while the pediatric head is for infants under the age of 2. For the standard head, its needles protrude 2 mm when the gun is actuated while for the pediatric heads, the needles protrude only 1 mm. Before application, the skin is cleaned with alcohol, then 100,000 units/ml (equivalent to about 0.1 ml) of tuberculin is evenly smeared on the skin and the gun applied to the skin and fired. The excess of the solution is then wiped off and a waterproof ink mark is drawn around the injection site as an indicator of the site of administration and the test read 2 to 7 days later. The results of the test are interpreted as follows:

Grade 0: no reaction, or induration of 3 or less puncture points;Grade 1: induration of four or more puncture points; Grade 2: induration of the six puncture points coalesce to form a circle; Grade 3: induration of 5 mm; or more and Grade 4: induration of 10 mm or more, or ulceration.

There is not much difference between the Heaf and Mantoux test, but the two tests can be related as follows: Heaf grade 0 and 1 approximately equivalent Mantoux less than 5 mm; Heaf grade 2 approximatley equivalent to Mantoux 5–14 mm and Heaf grade 3 & 4 being approximately equivalent to Mantoux 15 mm or greater, To avoid cases of false positives and false negatives, the tuberculin used for Heaf tests is 1000 times more concentrated than that used for Mantoux tests. In countries where both tests are used, use of the correct concentration avoids false positive and false negative results.

The recommended Tuberculin Skin Test (TST), which has now been standardised by the WHO to contain 0.1 ml of tuberculin (100 units/ ml), is the Mantoux test (CDC, 2010). The dosage of 0.1 ml containing 5 tuberculin units [TU] of purified protein derivative (PPD) should be injected intradermally into the volar aspect of the forearm using a 27-gauge needle. A detergent called Tween 80 to prevent loss of efficacy on contact and adsorption by glass stabilizes the PPD. A wheal should be raised and should measure approximately 6-10 mm in diameter. Skilled personnel should always read the test 48-72 hours after administration. Measure the amount of induration and not erythema. This should be measured transverse to the long axis of the forearm. Multiple puncture tests such as Tine test and Heaf test lack sensitivity and specificity and hence are not recommended in this situation (Marais et al., 2006).

Subcutaneous injection should be avoided because it results in false negative results. The site of administration is indicated by a water-proof ink mark drawn around the site of injection to serve as an indicator for the site. The reading, which is done two to seven days involves measuring area of induration transversely (left to right) across the forearm and recorded to the nearest millimetre. It should be borne in mind that the induration (dermal thickening causing the cutaneous surface to feel thicker and firmer) should not be confused with erythema (redness of the skin) caused by hyperemia of the capillaries in the lower layers of the skin.

If a patient who has previously had a negative tuberculin skin test develops a positive tuberculin skin test at a later date, tuberculin conversion is said to have occurred. When such a reaction occurs, it provides strong evidence for significant exposure to TB. Different countries have different standards about the time interval between tests. The UK recommendation is that the two tests have to be done at least six weeks apart; while in the U.S. the recommendation is that the two tests can be done one week apart.

Another phenomenon associated with tuberculin skin test is what is called boosting, which occurs when people who have had some traces of infection with M. tuberculosis and/or previous exposure to BCG vaccination against tuberculosis, are given repeated tuberculin skin tests. In these cases, the first test revives or primes the immune response so that on repeat testing, the response is much stronger and the patient now appears to have a positive reaction. The second tuberculin skin test result is what is taken to be the correct one. Again, the guidelines on how to approach the phenomenon of boosting are different in different countries with the U.S. guidelines emphasising that, ignoring previous immunisation with BCG would lead to a person showing the phenomenon of boosting, being falsely described as a tuberculin converter. On the other hand, UK guidelines advocate two tuberculin skin tests one week apart, if boosting is suspected, taking the result of the second test as being the true result. The phenomenon of boosting can occur up to two years after the first Mantoux test.

According to the American Academy of Pediatrics (AAP) immediate skin testing is indicated for the following children: 1)Those who have been in contact with persons with active or suspected TB; 2) Immigrants from TB-endemic countries or children with travel histories to these countries; 3) Those who have radiographic or clinical findings suggestive of TB. 4) Children who are infected with human immunodeficiency virus (HIV) or those living in a household with persons infected with HIV and; 5) Incarcerated adolescents.

Testing at 2-year to 3-year intervals is indicated if the child has been exposed to high-risk individuals including those who are homeless, institutionalized adults who are infected with HIV, users of illicit drugs, residents of nursing homes, and incarcerated adolescents or adults. Testing when children are aged 4-6 years and 11-16 years is indicated for the following children:1) Children without risk factors residing in high-prevalence areas; 2) Children whose parents emigrated from regions of the world with a high prevalence of TB or who have continued potential exposure by travel to the endemic areas and/or household contact. Performing an initial TST before the initiation of immunosuppressive therapy is recommended in any patient (AAP, 1996).

Wit regard to administering the TST to previous recipients of the Bacille Calmette-Guérin (BCG) several problems are encountered when it comes to interpreting the results of the test. Immunization with BCG is not a contraindication to the TST but differentiating tuberculin reactions caused by vaccination with BCG versus reactions caused by infection with M tuberculosis is difficult. History of contact with a person with contagious TB or emigration from a country with a high prevalence of TB suggests that the positive results are due to infection with M tuberculosis. However, multiple BCG vaccinations may increase the likelihood that the positive TST result is due to the BCG vaccination. The positive reactivity caused by BCG vaccination generally wanes with the passage of time. With the administration of TST, this positive tuberculin reactivity may be boosted. However, previous BCG vaccin not affect interpretation of a TST result for a person who is symptomatic or in whom TB is strongly suspected (Marais et al., 2006).

For the UK the guidelines for interpreting tuberculin skin tests are formulated according to the Heaf test. For patients who have had BCG previously, latent TB is diagnosed if the Heaf test is grade 3 or 4 and have no signs or symptoms of active; if the Heaf test is grade 0 or 1, then the test is repeated and, in patients who have not had BCG previously, latent TB isiag-nosed if the Heaf test if grade 2, 3 or 4, and have no signs or symptoms of active TB. Repeat Heaf testing is not done in patients who have had BCG of the phenomenon of boosting.

The Centers for Disease Control and Prevention (CDC) and the AAP provided recommenda-tions regarding the size of the induration created by the TST that is considered a positive result and indicative of disease [http://www.cdc.gov/tb/]. The TST is interpreted on the basis of 3 "cut points": 5 mm, 10 mm, and 15 mm. Induration of 5 mm or more is considered a positive TST result in the following children: 1) Children having close contact with known or suspected contagious cases of the disease, including those with household contacts with active TB whose treatment cannot be verified before exposure; 2) Children with immunosuppressive conditions (such as HIV) or children who are on immunosuppressive medications; 3) Children who have an abnormal chest radiograph finding consistent with active TB, previously active TB, or clinical evidence of the disease.

Induration of 10 mm or more is considered a positive TST result in the following children: 1) Children who are at a higher risk of dissemination of TB disease, including those younger than 5 years or those who are immunosuppressed because of conditions such as lymphoma, Hodgkin disease, diabetes mellitus, and malnutrition; 2) Children with increased exposure to the disease, including those who are exposed to adults in high-risk categories (such as homeless, HIV infected, users of illicit drugs, residents of nursing homes, incarcerated or institutionalized persons); 3) those who were born in or whose parents were born in high-prevalence areas of the world; and those with travel histories to high-prevalence areas of the world. Induration of 15 mm or more is considered a positive TST result in children aged 5 years or older without any risk factors for the disease.

False-positive reactions and false-negative results are common and can be due to various causes. False-positive reactions are often attributed to asymptomatic infection by environ-mental non-TB mycobacteria (due to cross-reactivity). False-negative results, on the other hand, may be due to vaccination with live-attenuated virus, anergy, immunosuppression, immune deficiency, or malnutrition. In cases of anergy, a lack of reaction by the body's defence mechanisms when it comes into contact with foreign substances, the tuberculin reaction will occur weakly, thus compromising the value of Mantoux testing. For example, anergy is present in AIDS, a disease which strongly depresses the immune system. Therefore, anergy testing is advised in cases where suspicion is warranted that it is present. However, routine anergy skin testing is not recommended. Other factors that may cause a false-negative result include improper administration (such as subcutaneous injection, injection of too little antigen), improper storage, and contamination. PPD has been recognized to have an initial false-negative rate of 29% (Marais et al., 2006).

With a TST, it is not possible to assert or deny the presence of TB, but it only indicates infection with a mycobacterium. In a child who has not been BCG-vaccinated, a TST has been defined as positive when the diameter of skin induration is greater than 10 mm, and in a BCG-vaccinated child, when the diameter of induration is greater than 15 mm. A negative TST does not exclude TB and some induration (5–14 mm) could be supportive if the clinical features and contact history are suggestive (Lewinsohn et al., 2004). Furthermore, the utility of this conventional test is hampered by technical and logistical problems: potential for false-positive and false-negative results; problems in administration and interpretation; difficulty in separating true infection from the effects of prior BCG vaccination, infection due to nontuberculous mycobacteria (Dogra et al., 2007). In children with debilitating or immunosuppressive illnesses, malnutrition, or viral (as HIV) and certain bacterial infections, the yield is unknown, but it is certainly higher than 10%. Moreover, false-positive reactions to TST are often attributed to asymptomatic infection by environmental nontuberculous mycobacteria (Nicol et al., 2011).

Given that the US guidelines recommend that previous BCG vaccination be ignored in the interpretation of tuberculin skin tests, false positives are possible. People who have previously had BCG, will falsely appear to be tuberculin converters and this may lead to treating more people than necessary, with the possible risk of those patients suffering adverse drug reactions. However, considering the fact that BCG vaccine is not 100% effective, and that it is less protective in adults than pediatric patients, not treating these patients could lead to a possible infection which tennds to justify the current US policy. The U.S. guidelines also allow for tuberculin skin testing in immunosuppressed patients whereas the UK guidelines recommend that tuberculin skin tests should not be used for such patients because it is unreliable

4.2. New approaches in TB diagnostics

4.2.1. Polymerase chain reaction (PCR)

Diagnostic PCR is a technique of in vitro DNA amplification that uses specific DNA sequences (oligonucleotides) as effective fishhooks for the DNA/cDNA of microorganisms. In theory, this technique can detect a single organism in a lot of specimens such as sputum, gastric aspirate, pleural fluid, cerebrospinal fluid, blood, and urine. Various PCR assays, mostly using the mycobacterial insertion element IS6110 as the DNA marker for M. tuberculosis-complex organisms, have a sensitivity and specificity greater than 90% for detecting pulmonary TB in adults. This is a rapid, sensitive, specific, and reasonable-cost (Montenegro et al., 2003) method for the detection of M. tuberculosis in clinical samples. The PCR may be used to (a) diagnose tuberculosis in difficult samples with negative microscopic examination, negative culture, or with scarce sample; (b) determine if the organisms in the sample are M. tuberculosis or atypical mycobacteria; (c) identify the presence of genetic variations like a mutations or deletions known to be associated with resistance to some antimycobacterial agents (Marais et al., 2005).

Studies in children have obtained better sensitivity by PCR than by culture. In 2001, Gomez-Pastrana et al., (2001) reported a comparison between sensitivity of culture and PCR showing higher sensitivity for the latter. PCR may have a special role in the diagnosis of extrapulmonary TB and pulmonary TB in children since sputum smears are usually unrevealing in these cases.

However, these tests are not performed correctly in all clinical laboratories. The cost involved, the need for sophisticated equipment, the limitations in their specificity, the need to obtain multiple samples to optimize yield and scrupulous technique to avoid cross-contamination of specimens preclude the use of PCR techniques in many developing countries (Montenegro et al., 2003).The sensitivity of PCR of gastric lavage/bronchoalveolar lavage has been found to be 56.8% in children with clinically active disease. Authors conclude that nested PCR is a rapid and sensitive method for the early diagnosis of TB in children. Additionally, other unique sequences of M. tuberculosis have been suggested as diagnostic test for TB, because they are absent in M. africanum, M. microti, M. bovis, and M. bovis BCG (Liang et al., 2008).

4.2.2. In-house nucleic acid amplification (NAA) assays

These assays are highly dependent on the operator's skills. Performance is also influenced by the choice of target sequence and DNA extraction method. Interpretation of the performance of these assays in pediatric TB suspects is hindered by the lack of a sensitive and specific reference standard. When compared with culture, the sensitivity of NAA for the diagnosis of childhood TB is typically low (40–83%). However, it appears, at least from some reports, that NAA identified a group of children who are clinically diagnosed with TB but in whom mycobacterial culture is negative. This means that with a proper technique it could be done efficiently (Nicol and Zar, 2011).

4.2.3. Adenosine deaminase

Adult studies have shown increased levels of adenosine deaminase (ADA) in pleural TB and TB-caused meningitis, both paucibacillary forms of TB, and have advocated for its use in diagnosis. Due to this evidence, a serum ADA has already been evaluated in a childhood population with a very high sensitivity (100%) and specificity (90.7%) for pulmonary TB. This study demonstrated the great potential of this technique because it has significant difference in serum ADA levels between children with disease and infection. However, there were several weaknesses in the study design, including unclear case definition, exclusion of nontuberculous patients, and a relatively small TB patient population (20 with active disease) (Marais. and Pai, 2007).

In the case of extrapulmonary TB, ADA measurement can be helpful, but its sensitivity and specificity varies widely and has been lower than multiplex PCR using primers for IS6110, dnaJ, and hsp65. Specifically, a meta-analysis of 63 studies of ADA in tuberculous pleuritis reveals that the sensitivity of the test is of 0.92 (95% CI 0.90–0.93) and specificity of 0.90 (95% CI 0.89–0.91) (Lawn and Nicol, 2011).

4.2.4. Serology and antigen detection

In absence of good diagnostic method for tuberculosis, the interest in serodiagnosis has been increased (Marais et al., 2005). Serological tests vary in a number of features, including antigen composition (38 kDa, Ag 60, and lipoarabinomannan, LAM), antigen source (native or recombinant), chemical composition (protein or lipid), extent of antigen(s) purification, and immunoglobulin detected. The majority are based on the enzyme-linked immunosorbent assay (ELISA) rapid versions and use various immunochromatographic formats, with lateral flow being the most popular.

A recent review of serological tests concluded that commercial antibody detection tests for extrapulmonary TB have no role in clinical care or case detection (Steingart et al., 2007). The search for novel biomarkers in blood or urine that can reliably distinguish active from latent TB in children with and without other co-infections remains an important global goal. Well-defined cohorts of paediatric patients in TB-endemic and non-endemic settings will be essential for initial screening and future validation of such potential markers. In the meantime, the diagnosis of TB in children in resource-poor countries continues to rely on practical algorithms, which lack standard symptom definitions and adequate validation (Marais et al., 2006). This poses an increased challenge in the context of HIV infection

Imaz et al., (2001) reported the importance of the recombinant 16-kDa antigen (re-Ag16) of M. tuberculosis in the serodiagnosis of tuberculosis (TB) in children measuring the values of IgA, IgM, and IgG and an increased mean antibody response to reAg16 was observed in contact children compared with nonmycobacterial disease patient with a 95% of specificity. A combining result of the IgG and IgA assays led to 43% positivity in children with active TB (Trilling. et al., 2011).

Mycobacterial antigen detection has been evaluated in adults, but rarely in children. Serology has found little place in the routine diagnosis of tuberculosis in children, even though it is rapid and does not require specimen from the site of disease. Sensitivity and specificity depend on the antigen used, gold standard for the diagnosis of tuberculosis, and the type of tubercular infection. Though most of these tests have high specificity, their sensitivity is poor because several factors can alter the results such as age, exposure to other mycobacteria, and BCG vaccination (Marais et al., 2005).

4.2.5. In vitro interferon-γ (IFN-γ) release assays (IGRAs) and antigen-testing

In addition to the traditional TST, which is known to lack both sensitivity and specificity, blood based assays have recently become available. These T-cell assays rely on stimulation of host blood cells with MTB specific antigens and measure production of IFN-γ. Numerous published studies compare the two available commercial assays, T Spot TB (Oxford Immunotec) and Quantiferon-Gold IT (Cellestis), with the TST for both detection of active disease and LTBI (Ferrara et al., 2006). T-cell assays have proven to be more specific than the TST, (Arend et al., 2007) but they are still unable to distinguish between active disease and LTBI. Interpretation therefore remains dependent on the clinical context. Some few studies have presented paediatric data but none have provided an assessment of age-related performance of these assays, and reservations remain regarding their performance in very young children and in immunocompromised populations, such as those with HIV (Clark et al., 2007).

There is still a lot of on going research aimed at establishing the proper role of gamma interferon tests and the guidelines ar still under constant review. The interferon-γ release assays (IGRAs) currently commercially available include QuantiFERON-TB Gold (QFT-G),

Quanti FERON-TB Gold In-Tube and T-SPOT.TB. These tests are aimed at he body's response to specific TB antigens not present in other forms of mycobacteria and BCG (ESAT-6). The tests are not affected by prior BCG vaccination, and despite their being new, these are now becoming available globally and CDC recommends that QFT-G may be used in all circumstances in which the TST is currently used, including contact investigations, evaluation of recent immigrants, and sequential-testing surveillance programs for infection control such as those for health-care workers. Health Protection Agency (HPA) recommends the use of IGRA testing in health care workers, if available, in view of the importance of detecting latently infected staff that may go on to develop active disease and come into contact with immunocompromised patients and the logistical simplicity of IGRA testing.

4.2.6. GeneXpert MTB/RIF system

GeneXpert includes the development of integrated DNA extraction and amplification systems. This requires minimal manipulation of sample and operator training. It utilizes real-time PCR (rt-PCR) technology to both diagnose TB and detect rifampicin resistance. The test amplifies a region of the rpoB gene of M. tuberculosis. Mutations of this region give rise to 95% of rifampicin resistance. Resistant strains contain mutations localized within the 81 bp core region of the bacterial RNA polymerase rpoB gene, which encodes the active site of the enzyme. In addition, the rpoB core region is flanked by Mycobacterium tuberculosis-specific DNA sequences. Thus, it is possible to test for M. tuberculosis and for rifampicin resistance simultaneously. The simplicity for the user makes this an assay that could feasibly be widely implemented outside centralized laboratories and potentially impacts on TB control (Gordet-sov et al., (2008). The Xpert system has some advantages over the cultivation, mainly in specificity and a shorter time to get results (Imaz. et al., 2001).

Recently, Nicol et al., (2011), reported the application of this method in 452 hospitalized children from South Africa, with or without HIV, with a median age of 19.4 months, and suspected of having TB. Two Xpert tests doubled the case detection rate compared with smear microscopy (76% versus 38%), identifying all smear-positive and 61% of smear-negative cases, the specificity was 98.8%. The sensitivities for smear-negative TB were 33.3% and 61.1% when testing one or two samples, respectively. The samplings were induced sputum and they detected three quarters of culture-confirmed tuberculosis with very high specificity; the yield of this method was twice that of smear microscopy. This could suggest the possibility of replacing the microscopy for this type of methodology which has greater sensitivity especially with a second sample (Rachow et al., 2011).

4.2.7. Gas sensor array electronic nose (electronic nose)

The potential to detect different Mycobacterium species in the headspaces of cultures and sputum samples is another innovative approach that is currently in development. The array uses 14 sensors to profile a "smell" by assessing the change in each sensor's electrical properties when exposed to a specific odour mixture. In an initial study using sputum samples from patients with culture-confirmed tuberculosis and those without tuberculosis, the E-Nose correctly predicted 89% of culture-positive patients with a specificity of 91% (Imaz. et al.,

2001). In a further development applying advanced data extraction and linear discriminant function analysis, obtained sensitivities were of 68% and 75%, and specificities of 75% and 67% for Rob and Walter electronic noses, respectively (Imaz. et al., 2001). Further applications of this test, including its potential value in the diagnosis of child tuberculosis, are needed.

4.3. Diagnosing congenital TB

Congenital TB is rare but symptoms typically develop during the second or third week of life and include poor feeding, poor weight gain, cough, lethargy, and irritability. Other symptoms include fever, ear discharge, and skin lesions. The principles in place are that for one to make a definitive diagnosis of congenital TB, the infant should have proven TB lesions and that it should have at least one of the following: 1) skin lesions during the first week of life, including papular lesions (ulcerated areas of the skin) or petechiae (bleeding into the skin); 2) documentation of TB infection of the placenta or the maternal genital tract; 3) presence of a primary complex in the liver and 4) the possibility of postnatal transmission should be ruled out. Signs of congenital TB include failure to thrive, icterus (jaundice or yellow skin), hepatosplenomegaly (enlargement of both the liver and spleen), tachypnea (rapid breathing), and lymphadenopathy (involving inflammation of lymphnodes) (Marais et al., 2006). Patients with asymptomatic infection have a positive tuberculin skin test (TST) result, but they do not have any clinical or radiographic manifestations. Children with asymptomatic infection may be identified on a routine healthy-child physical examination, or they may be identified subsequent to TB diagnosis in household or other contacts (for example, children who recently have immigrated or adopted children). Primary TB is characterized by the absence of any signs on clinical evaluation. As discussed above, these patients are identified by a positive TST result. Tuberculin hypersensitivity may be associated with erythema nodosum and phlyctenular conjunctivitis (Marais et al., 2006).

Endobronchial TB with lymphadenopathy, which is the disease with enlargement of lymph nodes, is the most common variety of pulmonary TB. Symptoms are the result of impingement on various structures by the enlarged lymph nodes. Enlargement of lymph nodes and persistent cough may result in signs suggestive of bronchial obstruction or hemi-diaphragmatic paralysis, whereas difficulty in swallowing may result from esophageal compression. Vocal cord paralysis may be suggested by hoarseness or difficulty breathing and may occur as a result of local nerve compression. Dysphagia (swallowing problems) due to esophageal compression may also be observed. Pleural effusions due to TB may also occur and usually occur in older children and are rarely associated with miliary disease. The typical history reveals an acute onset of fever, chest pain that increases in intensity on deep inspiration, and shortness of breath. Fever usually persists for 14-21 days. Signs include: tachypnea, respiratory distress, decreased breath sounds, and, occasionally, features of mediastinal shift (moving of the tissues and organs that comprise the mediastinum) (Marais et al., 2006).

Progression of the pulmonary parenchymal component of TB leads to enlargement of the caseous area (caseated = cheese-like necrotised tissue) and may lead to pneumonia, atelectasis (collapse of lung tissue), and air trapping. This is more likely to occur in young children than in adolescents. The child usually appears ill with symptoms of fever, cough, malaise, and weight loss. This condition presents with classic signs of pneumonia, including tachypnea, nasal flaring, grunting, dullness to percussion, egophony or egobronchophony (increased resonance of voice sounds, with a high-pitched bleating quality, heard especially over lung tissue compressed by pleural effusion); decreased breath sounds, and crackles (Marais et al., 2006). Reactivation of TB disease usually has a sub-acute presentation with weight loss, fever, cough, and, rarely, hemoptysis (coughing up of blood or bloody sputum from the lungs or airway). This condition typically occurs in older children and adolescent and is more common in patients who acquire TB at age 7 years and older. Physical examination results may be normal or may reveal post-tussive crackles (Marais et al., 2006).

4.4. Diagnosis of extrapulmonary TB

In this case the clinical picture is used to get an indication of the diagnosis. The diagnosis at any site should be confirmed by obtaining specimens for bacteriology wherever possible. This means that fluid aspirated or biopsies taken should be placed in a medium such as saline which will not kill the bacteria. Too often still biopsy specimens are placed in formalin so that bacteriological confirmation including sensitivity testing cannot be done. Miliary TB may manifest sub acutely with low-grade fever, malaise, weight loss, and fatigue. A rapid onset of fever and associated symptoms may also be observed. History of cough and respiratory distress may be obtained. Physical examination findings include lymphadenopathy, hepatos- plenomegaly, and systemic signs including fever. Respiratory signs may evolve to include tachypnea, cyanosis, and respiratory distress. Other signs, which are subtle and should be carefully sought in the physical examination, include papular, necrotic, or purpuric lesions on the skin or choroidal tubercles in the retina (Marais et al., 2006).

Patients with lymphadenopathy (scrofula or deposits in subcutaneous lymphatic ganglia) may have a history of enlarged nodes. Fever, weight loss, fatigue, and malaise are usually absent or minimal. One of the most severe complications of TB is TB meningitis, which develops in 5-10% of children younger than 2 years; thereafter, the frequency drops to less than 1%. A very high index of suspicion is required to make a timely diagnosis because of the insidious onset of the disease. A sub-acute presentation usually occurs within 3-6 months after the initial infection. Nonspecific symptoms such as anorexia, weight loss, and fever may be present. After 1-2 weeks, patients may experience vomiting and seizures or alteration in the sensorium (the part of the cerebral cortex that receives and coordinates all the impulses sent to individual nerve centers which includes auditory, gustatory, olfactory, somatosensory and visual centers). Deterioration of mental status, coma, and death may occur despite prompt diagnosis and early intervention.

Three stages of TB meningitis have been identified. Stage 1 is defined by the absence of focal or generalized neurologic signs. Possibly, only nonspecific behavioral abnormalities are found. Stage 2 is characterized by the presence of nuchal rigidity (inability or discomfort during neck flexion), altered deep tendon reflexes, lethargy (abnormal lack of energy), and/or cranial nerve palsies. TB meningitis most often affects the sixth cranial nerve due to the pressure of the thick basilar inflammatory exudates on the cranial nerves or to hydrocephalus; this results in lateral rectus palsy. The third, fourth, and seventh cranial nerves may also be affected. Funduscopic changes may include papilledema (swelling of the optic disc from increased intracranial pressure) and the presence of choroid tubercles (chroid plexus = vascular proliferation of the cerebral ventricles that serves to regulate intraventricular pressure by secretion or absorption of cerebrospinal fluid).which should be carefully sought. Stage 3, the final stage, comprises major neurologic defects, including coma, seizures, and abnormal movements such as choreoathetosis (irregular involuntary movements that may involve the face, neck, trunk, extremities, or respiratory muscles, giving an appearance of restlessness), paresis (slight or incomplete paralysis), paralysis of one or more extremities. In the terminal phase, decerebrate (elimination of cerebral brain function) or decorticate posturing, opisthotonus (a type of spasm in which the head and heels arch backward in extreme hyperextension and the body forms a reverse bow), and/or death may occur. Patients with tuberculomas or TB brain abscesses may present with focal neurologic signs. Spinal cord disease may result in the acute development of spinal block or a transverse myelitis–like syndrome (an abnormal condition characterized by inflammation of the spinal cord with associated motor or sensory dysfunction). A slowly ascending paralysis may develop over several months to years.

4.5. Treatment

4.5.1. General treatment overview

Each of the first-line drugs makes a specific contribution during different periods of drug action (assuming complete drug susceptibility and the absence of significant immune compromise). Period 1 lasts 2 to 3 days (van der Weert et al., 2006), during which time fast-growing extracellular bacilli, comprising the vast majority of the organism load, are killed, mainly by the excellent bactericidal activity of isoniazid (INH) (Kampmann et al., 2005). Period 2 lasts 4 to 8 weeks. Slower growing extracellular bacilli are killed (van der Weert et al., 2006) and the rate of killing is determined more by the physiological state of the bacilli and less by the bactericidal activity of the drug. During this period, the bactericidal activity of rifampin (RIF) is important and pyrazinamide (PZA) contributes by killing extracellular bacilli that persist in acidic areas of inflammation (van der Weert et al., 2006). Period 3 lasts 4 to 6 months. Persistent intracellular bacilli are eradicated mainly by RIF, although INH will continue to offer protection against the development of resistance and may assist with organism eradication, especially in fibrocaseous tissue with poor drug penetration. Host immunity plays an important role throughout, but is of particular importance to effect organism eradication and prevent disease relapse, as indicated by the high relapse rate in HIV-infected children.

Practical operational issues are extremely important for effective public health intervention. Operational issues include access to early and accurate diagnosis, the uninterrupted provision of quality-assured drugs and appropriate treatment regimens, as well as the establishment of systems to ensure good treatment adherence. Fixed-dose combinations should be used whenever possible to reduce the risk of drug resistance and to improve simplicity and adherence, but quality assurance is essential to ensure optimal bioavailability of all the constituent drugs (Dekker and Lotter, 2003). With proper implementation, the World Health Organization's directly observed therapy, short-course (DOTS) strategy addresses most of the important operational issues. However, the predominant emphasis of the DOTS strategy on sputum smear–positive disease excludes the vast majority of children. There is a desperate need to improve service delivery to children with tuberculosis, particularly in endemic areas with limited resources (Starke, 2002).

4.5.2. Preventive chemotherapy

Chemoprophylaxis refers to preventive treatment given after exposure (without proof of infection), whereas treatment of latent infection implies that infection (indicated by a positive TST) was documented. The term preventive chemotherapy is preferred because it is more inclusive and incorporates both chemoprophylaxis and treatment of latent infection. The TST is a fairly accurate measure of infection after exposure in immune-competent children, although TST conversion, which reflects a sufficiently strong delayed-type hypersensitivity response, may be delayed for up to 3 months (Marais et al., 2004). Therefore, household exposure, particularly involving high-risk children, should be treated as infection until the absence of infection can be convincingly demonstrated. In immune-competent children this can be done by repeating the TST 3 months after exposure ended (American Thoracic Society, 2000). In immunocompromised children the TST is not a sufficiently reliable test to exclude M. tuberculosis infection and children with documented exposure should receive preventive chemotherapy as if they are infected (Marais et al., 2006).

The reality on the ground is that most endemic areas do not have the capacity to follow current World Health Organization guidelines regarding the use of preventive chemotherapy in children, which advise active tracing and screening of all children less than 5 years old in household contact with a sputum smear–positive adult source case. This results mainly from the huge burden of adult tuberculosis and resource constraints that limit the ability to perform TST and chest X-ray screening tests. Because the TST and chest X-ray are regarded as prerequisite screening tests, screening of exposed children and the provision of preventive chemotherapy are not even attempted in most resource-constrained areas. Access to preventive chemotherapy in these settings may be improved by employing symptom-based screening, although the benefits and risks of such a simplified approach require further evaluation. A study from an endemic area indicated that symptom-based screening may identify those children who require further investigation to exclude active tuberculosis (Marais et al., 2006), thus allowing asymptomatic household contacts, especially those who are at high risk to progress to disease, immediate access to preventive therapy despite the inability to perform TST and chest X-ray–based screening (Marais et al., 2006).

Another consideration is that in some endemic areas the majority of disease transmission, particularly in children greater than 2 to 3 years of age, occurs outside the household (Verver et al., 2004). In endemic areas, narrowing the focus of contact tracing to those children who are at highest risk to progress to disease after exposure or infection (less than 3 years of age and/or immune compromised) will decrease the burden placed on already overstretched health care systems, while still ensuring access to preventive chemotherapy for the children who need it most (Van Zyl et al., 2006). In older (greater than 3 years of age), immune-competent children the risk of tuberculosis after exposure is low and disease progression is usually indicated by the presence of persistent, slowly progressive symptoms. Therefore, passive case finding together with adequate diagnostic vigilance seems appropriate in this low-risk group.

In non endemic areas where resources permit and where the risk of future reinfection is low, it seems warranted to extend preventive chemotherapy to low-risk children as well, to eliminate the reservoir of latent infection within the community. INH monotherapy for 6 to 9 months is the best-studied chemoprophylactic regimen and it reduces the tuberculosis risk in exposed children by at least two-thirds; probably by more than 90% with good adherence. However, poor adherence is a major concern, particularly in endemic areas (Van Zyl et al., 2006).

In real life the effectiveness of a preventive chemotherapy regimen is determined first by its efficacy and second by adherence to the prescribed regimen. Because of documented poor adherence to 6–9 months of unsupervised INH monotherapy, consideration should be given to alternative preventive strategies with comparable efficacy but with improved adherence. Theoretically the addition of RIF has important advantages; RIF has strong sterilizing activity to eradicate latent bacilli and its addition will shorten the duration of treatment required (Mitchison, 2005). It will also improve efficacy in settings where INH mono-resistance is prevalent. The use of a 3-month INH and RIF regimen for preventive chemotherapy is well established and trials have shown equivalence to 6 to 9 months of INH alone, although the evidence is not as comprehensive as that for INH monotherapy (Ena and Valls, 2005).

PZA is another important sterilizing drug and in theory the combination of RIF and PZA represents the treatment of choice for latent infection. This combination has proven efficacy in animal but adverse reactions in adults have limited the initial enthusiasm (Priest, 2004). However, these adverse reactions have not been observed in children, in whom the three-drug combination of INH, RIF, and PZA is generally well tolerated (Marais et al., 2006). Adherence may be improved by shortening the duration of treatment, but consideration may also be given to the provision of supervised preventive therapy. Creative approaches will be required to achieve this, particularly in places where health care services are already overburdened. With curative treatment, intermittent (two or three times weekly) therapy during the continuation phase is as effective as daily therapy to achieve organism eradication, once the organism load has been sufficiently reduced (Al-Dossary et al., 2002). The same principle would apply to the treatment of latent infection, where the organism load is low. Targeting high-risk children for short-course, supervised intermittent preventive therapy seems achievable, but defining optimal preventive therapy regimens remains a fertile and important area for future research (Marais et al., 2006).

Vaccination with BCG is the most widely used preventive strategy, although its efficacy remains controversial and studies have shown that it contributes to this variable protection: variations in strain-specific immunogenicity, timing and technique of vaccine administration, genetic factors, the presence or absence of environmental mycobacteria, and the effect of multiple re-infection events as may occur in highly endemic areas. It is generally accepted that BCG vaccination offers significant protection against disseminated disease in young children (below 2 years), but that it offers little or no protection against adult-type tuberculosis.

However, reports have documented significant protection against the development of adult-type tuberculosis when BCG was administered to TST-negative adolescents in locations with a low prevalence of environmental mycobacterial exposure (Bjarveit et al., 2003).

In addition, a report from Turkey indicated that contrary to the prevailing theory, BCG may also protect against M. tuberculosis infection as based on a positive enzyme-linked immuno-spot result. An even more controversial area is the risk versus benefit that BCG provides to HIV-infected children. There is a definite risk for HIV-infected infants to develop severe forms of BCG disease after neonatal BCG vaccination (Hesseling et al., 2006), but it remains poorly quantified. As the risk:benefit ratio has not been determined, the World Health Organization still advises BCG vaccination of asymptomatic HIV-exposed infants in tuberculosis endemic areas. Establishing the risk: benefit ratio of BCG vaccination in HIV-infected infants and the development of novel vaccines with improved efficacy and safety, remain major research challenges (Marais et al., 2006).

4.5.3. Curative treatment

The main variables that influence the success of chemotherapy, apart from primary drug resistance, are the bacterial load and the anatomic distribution of bacilli. Cavitary disease indicates a high bacterial load, as demonstrated by the frequency with which these patients are sputum smear–positive, which implies an increased risk for random drug resistance against individual drugs. Disseminated disease may signify penetration of bacilli into the central nervous system (CNS) (Van den Bosch et al., 2004) implying that adequate drug penetration across the blood–brain barrier is an important requirement for the treatment of disseminated disease (Marais et al., 2006).

From a public health perspective the challenge is to develop a pragmatic classification of childhood tuberculosis that incorporates the diverse spectrum of disease, but focuses primarily on treatment relevance. The main variables that influence the success of chemotherapy identify three groups of children with tuberculosis: (1) those with sputum smear–negative disease, (2) those with sputum smear–positive (often cavitary) disease and (3) those with disseminated disease. The discussion reflects current treatment guidelines for these three groups as well as the new regimens to consider on the basis of established treatment principles (Marais et al., 2006).

As a guide for individual patient classification and management five simple questions have been formulated: (1) Is the child exposed to or infected with M. tuberculosis? (2) Does the child have active tuberculosis? (3) If the child is exposed or infected, but does not have active tuberculosis, is preventive chemotherapy indicated? (4) If the child has active tuberculosis, what is the appropriate treatment regimen? (5) Are there any special circumstances such as HIV infection, retreatment, or exposure to a drug-resistant source case to consider? The underlying rationale is universally applicable irrespective of diagnostic or resource constraints; although areas with access to advanced technology may achieve improved levels of diagnostic certainty.

Sputum smear–negative disease is usually paucibacillary and therefore the risk of acquired drug resistance is low. Drug penetration into the anatomic sites involved is good and the success of three drugs (INH, RIF, and PZA) during the 2-month intensive phase, and of two drugs (INH and RIF) during the 4-month continuation phase, is well established. In the presence of extensive radiographic disease with or without cavitation, and/or suspicion of INH resistance, the use of ethambutol (EMB) in addition to the three drugs during the intensive phase should be contemplated. After completion of the intensive phase, successful organism eradication may be achieved with intermittent (two or three times weekly) therapy during the continuation phase (Al-Dossary et al., 2002). The efficacy of shorter treatment durations for HIV-uninfected immune-competent children with sputum smear–negative disease requires further evaluation, as a 4-month regimen of INH and RIF may be an acceptable therapy for some adults with sputum smear– and culture-negative tuberculosis.

Sputum smear–positive disease implies a high organism load and an increased risk for random drug resistance against individual drugs. Selecting drug-resistant mutants is a particular concern where INH mono-resistance is prevalent, as this increases the likelihood of selecting multidrug-resistant (MDR) organisms. The use of four drugs (INH, RIF, PZA, and EMB) during the 2-month intensive phase should reduce this risk. Once the organism load is sufficiently reduced, intermittent (two or three times weekly) therapy with INH and RIF during the 4-month continuation phase is sufficient to ensure organism eradication (Al-Dossary et al., 2002). However, caution should be exercised when initial treatment response has not been optimal and in HIV-infected patients. The use of long-acting rifamycins together with INH is discouraged (Rieder et al., 2001).

Disseminated disease is frequently associated with CNS involvement (Donald et al., 2005). It is therefore essential to consider the cerebrospinal fluid (CSF) penetration of drugs used in the treatment of disseminated disease. INH and PZA penetrate the CSF well. RIF and streptomycin penetrate the CSF poorly, but may achieve therapeutic levels in the presence of meningeal inflammation. The value of streptomycin is limited by poor CSF penetration and intramuscular administration. EMB hardly penetrates the CSF, even in the presence of meningeal inflammation, and has no demonstrated efficacy in the treatment of TBM. Ethionamide shows good CSF penetration and has been used successfully as a fourth drug in the treatment of TBM. The fact that RIF penetrates the CSF poorly in the absence of meningeal inflammation reduces its sterilization value and may warrant the inclusion of PZA during the continuation phase, to assist with CNS sterilization.

Several reports have illustrated the efficacy of short-course regimens in the treatment of TB meningitis, but the risk of CNS relapse is rarely reported. In two of these studies a relapse was documented despite the completion of 6 months of treatment with INH and RIF with an initial 2 months of PZA. Therefore, it seems prudent to include a fourth drug with good CNS penetration (such as ethionamide) for the treatment of disseminated disease, at least during the intensive phase, and to consider PZA for the full 6 months of treatment to reduce the risk of CNS relapse. CNS relapse is rare in the United States, where PZA is routinely discontinued after 2 months, but the total treatment duration is 9 to 12 months. Current fixed-dose combination tablets provide 4 to 6 mg of INH per kilogram. This dose may be suboptimal, particularly in settings where the majority of the bacterial population rapidly acetylates INH (Schaaf et al., 2005). In addition, the serum level achieved with a similar dose of INH per kilogram is lower in children than in adults, increasing the risk for suboptimal dosing in children (Schaaf et al., 2005). The majority of new INH resistance encountered in endemic areas is of an intermediate or low level, which underscores the importance of optimal INH dosing (Donald et al., 2004). A standard INH dose of 10 mg/kg seems appropriate in children, as even doses up to 20 mg/kg are well tolerated (Schaaf et al., 2005); children are less susceptible to the toxic effects of INH than are adults.

In general, adverse events are less common in children than in adults. The most severe adverse event is the development of hepatotoxicity, which can be caused by INH, RIF, PZA, or ethionamide. An elevation of liver enzymes (less than five times normal values) is not an indication to stop treatment, but the occurrence of liver tenderness, hepatomegaly, or jaundice should prompt the immediate stopping of all potentially hepatotoxic drugs. Jaundice is often preceded by a period of days or weeks of malaise and nausea. Hepatic reactions usually occur in the first weeks of therapy, but may happen at any time during the treatment period. Drug-related hepatic toxicity is usually caused by a single drug, but rarely a combination of drugs, which individually cause no problem, may cause hepatic toxicity. Children should be screened for other causes of hepatitis, as in many cases the anti-tuberculosis drugs are not the cause of liver function derangement. In South Africa, hepatitis A infection is frequently responsible for non–drug-related liver function derangement in children receiving anti-tuberculosis treatment. Potentially hepatotoxic drugs should be reintroduced only after liver functions have normalized. Non-hepatotoxic drugs should be used in the interim and expert opinion should be sought.

Ethambutol is usually not advised in children less than 7 years as visual acuity cannot be evaluated. However, its use may be warranted in children with hepatotoxicity, cavitary disease, or resistance to first-line drugs; it seems safe at recommended dosages. Ethionamide frequently causes vomiting, but this can usually be overcome by dividing the daily dose and by a slow increase up to the full dose during the first week or two of therapy. Recommended dosages for the various first- and second-line drugs are reflected in the publication by Marais et al., (2006) as indicated in the Table 1 below:

Despite significant symptomatic improvement radiographic disease resolution may take many months; persistent radiographic signs are not an indication to change treatment if there is clinical improvement. Paradoxical exacerbation of symptoms or signs may also occur after anti-tuberculosis therapy is initiated. This results from immune reconstitution with increased inflammation, particularly surrounding diseased lymph nodes or tuberculomas, that may follow nutritional rehabilitation (Marais et al., 2004), and/or antiretroviral therapy. The release of bacterial toxins after successful anti-tuberculosis treatment may also contribute.

Treatment should be continued unaltered, although the temporary addition of corticosteroids may be considered. Such adjunctive therapy may be helpful in a number of disease manifestations where the host inflammatory response contributes to disease pathology such as CNS involvement, severe lymph node compression of the airways, and pericardial effusion. There

		Maximum Dosage (mg/kg/dose)	
	Mode of Action	Daily	Two or Three Times/wk
First-line drugs			
Isoniazid	Bactericidal	10–15 (300 mg)	20–30 (900 mg)
Rifampin	Bactericidal and sterilizing	10–20 (600 mg)	10–20 (600 mg)
Pyrazinamide	Sterilizing	20–40 (2,000 mg)	50 (2,000 mg)
Ethambutol	Bacteriostatic	15–25 (1,200 mg)	30–50 (2,500 mg)
Second-line drugs			
Ethionamide or prothionamide	Bactericidal	15–20 (1,000 mg)	NA
Streptomycin	Bacteriostatic	20–40 (1,000 mg)	NA
Fluoroquinolones	Bactericidal		NA
Ciprofloxacin		20–40 (1,500 mg)	
Aminoglycosides	Bacteriostatic		NA
Kanamycin		15–30 (1,000 mg)	
Amikacin		15–30 (1,000 mg)	
Capreomycin		15–30 (1,000 mg)	
Cycloserine or terizidone	Bacteriostatic	10–20 (1,000 mg)	NA
Para-aminosalicylic acid	Bacteriostatic	200–300 (10 g)	NA

NA = not applicable. Source: Marais et al., (2006).

Table 1. First- And Second-Line Antituberculosis Drugs And Recommended Dosages In Children

is insufficient evidence to demonstrate whether steroids are effective in tuberculous pleural effusion.

4.5.4. Retreatment

Anti-tuberculosis treatment rarely fails in children and, if it does, every effort should be made to find the most likely cause. In settings where the prevalence of drug resistance is low the commonest cause is failure to properly take the medications, which can occur even during DOT, if supervision is not complete. It is important to remember that non-adherence has a differential diagnosis; there are psychologic, sociologic, religious, economic, and practical reasons why people are non-adherent and one must deal with all these issues for chemotherapy to be successful. With treatment interruption the child may be restarted on the original treatment regimen while ensuring adequate supervision, as the risk of developing drug resistance is small in children with paucibacillary disease. If an immune-competent child presents with a new episode of tuberculosis more than 6 months after completing treatment for a previous episode, then it most likely represents re-infection disease and standard first-line treatment is appropriate. In the case of genuine treatment failure (absence of clinical response to supervised treatment) drug susceptibility testing is of paramount importance. If an adult source case is identified with drug-resistant tuberculosis, the child should be treated according to the drug susceptibility pattern of the source case's strain (Marais et al., 2006).

4.5.5. Treatment of paediatric TB/HIV co-infection

The high risk of HIV-infected children to progress to disease after infection justifies the use of preventive chemotherapy in children who are latently infected. However, the difficult issue in endemic areas is how to deal with the ever-present risk of undocumented re-infection within the community. The prevention or reversal of severe immune compromise by using highly active antiretroviral therapy (HAART) should preclude the need for repeated or continuous preventive chemotherapy, although the risk for tuberculosis probably remains higher than in HIV-uninfected children. The cellular immune response assists with organism eradication and therefore it is not unexpected that disease relapse has been documented in HIV-infected children. The value of prolonging the treatment duration from 6 to 9 months, to ensure organism eradication in HIV-infected children, is under investigation. During a repeat episode both relapse and reinfection should be considered and every effort should be made to establish a culture-confirmed diagnosis and to do drug susceptibility testing (Marais et al., 2006).

When initiating treatment (curative treatment or RIF-containing preventive therapy) in HIV-infected children already receiving HAART or for whom HAART is contemplated, it should be appreciated that the rifamycins, especially RIF, and some of the nonnucleoside reverse transcriptase inhibitors and/or protease inhibitors may cause significant drug interactions. HIV-infected children may also develop particularly pronounced paradoxical reactions after the institution of HAART, because of immune reconstitution inflammatory syndrome. Recommendations on optimal drug combinations are frequently revised. The most recent recommendations can be obtained from the Centers for Disease Control and Prevention website, at [http://www.cdc.gov/nchstp/tb/].

Latest WHO recommendations advise starting antiretroviral therapy (ART) once anti-TB therapy (ATT) is established (after a period of 2-8 weeks) for all WHO clinical Stage Four HIV-infected children and Stage Three children with advanced or severe immunosuppression. For children in WHO clinical stage with mild or no immunosuppression, ART may be deferred until 6 months of ATT are completed (WHO, 2006). On-going prospective trials involving adults and children in TB/HIV endemic countries might provide future guidelines for the ideal timing of the initiation of anti-retroviral therapy (ART) in patients with HIV receiving TB therapy. There is already evidence from prospective trials that shows that high mortality is associated with TB in advanced stages of HIV-disease in children who do not receive ART promptly. Further research is required to improve our understanding of immune reconstitution disease (IRD) in children (Walters et al., 2006). Also, therapeutic drug monitoring (TDM), where available, should be undertaken when children are receiving concomitant ART and ATT. TDM data from ethnically similar children in resource-rich countries may in the future inform dosing recommendations in resource-poor settings where TDM is not available.

4.5.6. Treatment of extrapulmonary paeditric PTB

Treatment is as for pulmonary disease, with isoniazid, rifampicin, pyrazinamide and etham-butol for two months followed by isoniazid and rifampicin for four months, except for CNS disease when treatment should be continued for a full year. Steroids may be used in pericardial and meningeal disease. Surgery is usually unnecessary, especially where lymph glands and abscess are present, as long term discharging sinuses may result. Surgery is sometimes necessary in spinal TB where there is instability and may be needed to overcome strictures in genito-urinary or gastro-intestinal disease. Occasionally pericardectomy may be required when pericardial disease causes tamponade.

4.5.7. Treatment of latent paediatric TB infection

Treatment of LTBI, also known as chemoprophylaxis, is important to prevent future disease activation. The fact that over 50% of hospitalized children with culture-confirmed TB have a reported close TB contact and do not receive chemoprophylaxis, is an indication of the important missed opportunities using existing public health interventions. For the last 20 years the WHO guidelines recommended all children under 5 years in close contact with an infectious (usually smear positive) case receive 6 months isoniazid. Once active disease has been excluded, isoniazid monotherapy for 6-9 months has been proven to reduce the TB risk in exposed children by over 90% with good adherence. More recent studies suggest that 3 months of combined isoniazid and rifampicin are equally effective (Ena and Valls, 2005). In a recent study with very short follow-up, continuous isoniazid prophylaxis for HIV-infected children without documented evidence of latent infection, but living in an environment of high exposure, has also been shown to reduce overall morbidity and mortality from TB and other infections (Zar et al., 2007). Further trials in HIV-infected children receiving ART are ongoing.

Recommendations for chemoprophylaxis will continue to differ in TB-endemic and non-endemic settings, because of the perceived risk of exposure. Whilst most paediatricians in Europe and North America would advocate chemoprophylaxis for HIV infected, TB-exposed children only, this needs to be interpreted with caution if the exposure is potentially ongoing or recurrent, and the ability to distinguish LTBI from active disease is limited. In this context, many practitioners in TB-endemic settings are reluctant to place children on chemoprophylaxis because of the potential emergence of resistant strains, if indeed the child has active disease instead of LTBI.

4.5.8. Treatment of drug resistant paediatric TB

Acquisition of resistance rarely occurs in children due to the paucibacillary nature of their disease but overall, children may also be subject to less selection pressure from anti TB therapy. Thus most resistance in children is due to primary transmission of a resistant organism, and MDR /XDR-TB rates in children reflect community transmission rates. Diagnosis requires a high index of suspicion as the culture yield in children makes definitive microbiological confirmation difficult. Resistance should be suspected if an index case has known resistant TB; the child shows initial improvement on anti-TB therapy and then deteriorates; or there is no response to initial treatment. Acquired resistance is well described in HIV co-infected adults previously treated for TB, possibly due to malabsorption of anti-TB drugs (Wells, et al., 2007). The presence of acquired resistance in the paediatric population is reported and in particular children with TB/HIV co-infection should be closely monitored (Soeters et al., 2005).

Although the principles of DOTS Plus have been put forward for the management of MDR TB, at the moment, there is no consensus for any regimen or optimal treatment that should be used for persons with known exposure to MDR-TB. The recommendation by CDC is a combination of pyrazinamide and ethambutol, with either pyrazinamide or a fluoroquinolone and that immunocompetent contacts should be treated for 6 months while immunocompro-mised contacts should be treated for 12 months. Current guidelines recommend using at least four drugs to which the patient is naïve, including an injectable and a fluoroquinolone, in an initial phase of at least 6 months; followed by at least three of the most active and best tolerated drugs in a 12-18 month continuation phase.

Standardised regimens have been developed for settings where drug susceptibility testing is not available (WHO, 2006). Six classes of second-line drugs (SLDs) are available (WHO, 2003) but experience in children is limited for the majority and multi-centre paediatric trials are needed. Under optimum circumstances MDR-TB responds well to appropriate therapy. However delays in diagnosis and treatment, adherence issues, and a lack of child-friendly formulations and strategies for DOTS all frequently complicate management and contribute to a high morbidity and mortality (Drobac et al., 2006).

The WHO currently recommends avoidance of chemoprophylaxis in cases of contact with known MDR-TB and to observe for 2 years if clinically asymptomatic. Children with latent MDR-TB infection become the reservoir for future transmission following disease reactivation in adulthood, emphasizing the need to further research and improved management of MDR-TB infection in children, both at the clinical and operational level.

According to the European Centre for Disease Prevention and Control (ECDC) 2012 Guide-lines, there are two valid options to consider for the management of MDR TB and XDR TB contacts; preventive treatment or follow-up by careful clinical observation. The purpose of preventive therapy is to prevent the progression of LTBI to TB disease in an individual who has been exposed to MDR/XDR TB. The concept of preventive therapy has been shown to be effective for LTBI after contact with drug-susceptible TB but corresponding evidence for preventive therapy of MDR TB and XDR TB contacts is very scarce. Although for children there are indications of a positive effect of preventive therapy, for other groups of contacts, the necessary body of evidence has yet to be generated, and there are ongoing studies to collect evidence in support of the use of preventive therapy in contacts of MDR TB cases.

There is currently no evidence available on the optimal follow-up time in contacts of MDR TB or XDR TB with regard to patient benefits and costs of the intervention. In young children under five years of age the majority (over 90%) of TB disease will devel-op within 12 months of infection. Infants and children under five years of age, immuno-compromised individuals due to HIV infection or TNF-antagonist treatment are at increased risk of progression from LTBI to TB disease. These individuals as well as other identified risk groups require special attention as part of the individual risk assessment (WHO, 2007; Salgado and Solovic et al., 2010).

The optimal duration of MDR-TB treatment in children is not known. World Health Organization guidelines recommend treatment until 18 months after the first negative culture (24 months in XDR-TB). As children often have paucibacillary disease, documenting a culture conversion is usually difficult. Thus, the same duration as in adults would apply. The duration of the intensive phase of treatment (when an injectable drug is given) should be at least 6 months. Surgical resection should be considered when the patient has localized lesions and has persistently positive smear or culture results inspite of aggressive chemotherapy (Shah, 2012).

4.5.9. BCG vaccination and HIV infection

Approaches for prevention of TB include prevention of infection (through immunization) or of progression from latent infection to disease (chemoprophylaxis). Bacille Calmette-Guérin (BCG) vaccine, a live attenuated vaccine derived from Mycobacterium bovis that was developed in the 1920s, is administered to children at birth in many countries. WHO guidelines recommend administration of BCG soon after birth to all infants in countries with a high TB prevalence. Current WHO guidelines advise that all children below 5 years of age, who are in close contact with a sputum smear-positive index patient, should be actively traced, screened for TB, and provided preventive chemotherapy after active TB has been excluded (Marais et al., 2004).

Although this is good policy, implementation is fraught with challenges, including difficulty in diagnosing latent TB in a highly BCG-vaccinated population, ruling out incipient active disease, and the lack of procedures for documentation and follow-up of contact screening and chemoprophylaxis in national programs. Because the majority of transmission in children below 3 years of age occurs in the household and they are also the group at highest risk of progression to disease after primary infection, this activity should be given higher priority in national infection-control programs. Moreover, active tracing and screening of household contacts at high risk would allow children with disease to receive a diagnosis earlier, thus reducing complications.

Furthermore, additional protection by revaccination with BCG has not been demonstrated (Rodrigues et al., 2005). To date, the efficacy of the BCG vaccination has not been determined in HIV infected individuals in whom the immune responses to BCG may be reduced, (Hesseli et al., 2007) although this is the subject of ongoing trials. Due to the risk of disseminated BCG disease which may rarely complicate use of this live vaccine in immunocompromised individuals, BCG vaccination is no longer recommended in children known to be HIV-infected (Hesseling et al., 2007). In practice, this has had little impact in HIV-endemic countries, where the HIV-status of the baby is rarely established at birth, the usual time of BCG vaccination.

A large trial in southern India that included over 350,000 participants aged above 1 year concluded that BCG vaccine did not offer protection against the development of adult pulmonary TB (WHO, 2006). However, BCG vaccine has been shown to be protective against disseminated forms of TB in young children, with a protective estimate ranging from 67%–79% against TB meningitis and 58%–87% against miliary disease. A theoretical model estimated that a universal BCG vaccine program would have a beneficial impact in settings with prevalence rates of greater than 30 sputum smear-positive cases/100,000 population (WHO, 2007). However, there is no evidence of any BCG-induced protective effect in HIV-infected children. On the contrary, studies have documented BCG-induced disseminated disease and adverse reactions. Therefore, the WHO recommendations have been revised, making HIV infection a contraindication for BCG vaccination, even in settings where TB is highly endemic. Strategies required for effective implementation of this policy change include high uptake of maternal HIV testing coupled with implementation of proven strategies to prevent mother-to-child HIV transmission, including maternal treatment with HAART and early virological diagnosis of HIV infection in infants, followed by treatment.

The revised recommendations present a dilemma for national programs. Although the benefits of BCG vaccine far outweigh the risk among HIV-uninfected children living in high areas with a high prevalence of TB, the risk is higher among HIV-infected infants with or without symptoms at the time of vaccination. National recommendations will need to consider a variety of factors, including the prevalence of TB in the population, the prevalence of HIV infection, the availability of HIV testing and facilities for prevention of mother-to-child transmission during pregnancy, the capacity to conduct follow-up of vaccinated children, and the availability of early infant diagnosis of HIV infection. Abandoning the use of BCG vaccine before newer vaccines become available may put millions of young children at risk of TB. There is an urgent need for operational research in TB endemic countries to determine the best way to manage this issue programmatically.

5. On-going research targeting paediatric TB

5.1. New vaccine pipelines

The global commitment of the WHO and the Stop TB (WHO, 2005) campaign has spurred on the efforts of the international research community to develop a more effective anti-TB vaccine by the year 2015. In view of the proven efficacy of existing BCG vaccine in preventing disseminated TB in children and reducing child mortality (Roth et al., 2006) two conceptually different strategies have been pursued: firstly, the development of 'priming vaccines', which, it is hoped, will replace BCG by providing better and longer protection; secondly, the design of 'booster vaccines' to boost pre-existing BCG-derived immunity. Novel vaccines currently under development all use a "booster-strategy" after priming with BCG in infancy (Doherty et al, 2007). As the current candidates are progressing through phase I and II trials, including studies in HIV-infected individuals and age-de-escalation, it is most likely that more than one vaccine will progress into phase III.

The most advanced vaccine candidate is MVA- 85A, currently in phase II under a prime-boost strategy with BCG. Four products are in phase I (72f, Hybrid 1, Aeras 402, rBCG-UreC-Hly), each stemming from PPPs. Many of the candidates are results from the EU FP6 projects, i.e.

TBVAC and Muvapred, where valuable progress has been achieved. Several other candidates are still in the pre-clinical phase. For example, mutation of virulence genes produced a TB strain potentially conferring greater protection with fewer side effects than BCG. In addition, an improved, recombinant BCG vaccine with a higher efficacy and a better safety profile moving into phase I clinical trials is a possible prospect.

New research is directed at the development of a multistage TB vaccine containing latency antigens, an attractive concept, which is actively being pursued (Andersen, 2007). Such a vaccine could be used as a booster vaccine with the goal of preventing new infections in those uninfected with MTB and to prevent reactivation in those with LTBI. Unfortunately, the lack of reliable correlates of protective immunity currently remains a major obstacle to predict vaccine efficacy in all TB vaccine trials for both adults and children.

6. Existing research gaps

6.1. Research needs

Tracing of MDR TB contacts is important to prevent TB disease and further transmission. Priority studies needed include those to identify the most effective contact-tracing procedures for close contacts and the most effective follow-up procedures in healthcare workers constantly exposed to MDR TB. As part of the management of MDR TB contacts, studies on specific groups are needed, for example on children below the age of five years, children with HIV infection and other immunocompromised states. In particular, studies are needed: 1) for treated contacts: (randomised) clinical trials: 2) to determine which drugs and which drug combinations and dosages are optimal for preventive therapy; 3) to determine the duration of preventive therapy; 4) to assess the effectiveness of preventive therapy in conjunction with antiretroviral treatment; 5) to assess the risk of development of new drug resistance in contacts receiving (inadequate and adequate) preventive therapy; 6) for untreated contacts, and healthcare workers constantly exposed to MDR TB: 7) to identify the optimal follow-up period for different groups of individuals; and 8) to identify the optimal frequency of testing for LTBI during the follow-up period.

In order to increase adherence to treatment of MDR/XDR TB contacts (and reduce the risk of development of new drug resistance in contacts), studies are needed: 1) to identify new drugs with less adverse events and to explore possible (positive and negative) interactions between combined drugs; 2) to identify biomarkers indicating the risk of progression from LTBI to TB disease and 3) to assess operational management to shorten preventive therapy. Since the provision of preventive therapy has economic and logistic implications at the national and community level, cost-effectiveness and cost-benefit studies are also needed. These studies are particularly valuable because they can help to inform the decision on intervention policies..

A substantial amount of funding has been injected into research on various aspects of TB but there are still many issues that require additional research especially in the area of childhood tuberculosis. The most salient ones include:1) accurately quantifying the global burden of childhood tuberculosis especially in the endemic areas; 2) improving the understanding of the disease interactions with the immune system and re-evaluating the role of BCG and the new vaccine candidates in protecting children and adults against TB; 3) defining the diagnostic contribution of novel T-cell–based assays in endemic and non-endemic areas especially with regard to diagnosis of paediatric tuberculosis; 4) identifying new ways of diagnosing childhood tuberculosis in HIV negative and in TB/HIV co-infection in children, particularly in resource-limited settings; 5) carrying out operational research aimed at improving the access of children in endemic areas to preventive therapy and treatment, using the existing DOTS/ DOTS Plus frameworks; 6) evaluating the efficacy of new short-course intermittent preventive chemotherapy regimens especially those aimed at childhood TB; 7) exploring shorter durations of treatment in immune-competent children with smear-negative disease; 8) defining the optimal treatment regimen and treatment duration in children with TB/HIV co-infection; 9) monitoring the impact of MDR and XDR tuberculosis on children and evaluating regimens for effective MDR/XDR disease prevention and treatment; 10) developing and evaluating new drugs that may shorten the treatment duration and/or assist with the treatment of MDR/XDR disease and emphasizing case finding and reporting as some of the strategies to combat the escalation of XDR-TB [http://ec.europa.eu/research/research-eu].

6.2. Need for more specific diagnostic tests

In the field of diagnosis, there is an urgent need to replace sputum microscopy the current gold standard test, with more sensitive tests that are applicable at point of care. Despite the fact that the technique can only pick up 60% of cases, it has been in use for over a hundred years. Furthermore, sputum culture is not suitable for extrapulmonary TB and for paediatric TB since children can not produce sputum. On the other hand, the newer immunological based tests such as IGRAs are not well suited for use in TB/HIV co-infection and in high burden TB areas, where they cannot be accurately used to distinguish active from latent TB. Since the majority of the infected people never actually develop the disease, there is need to have a diagnostic tool which is able to distinguish latent from active disease and help to identify healthy individuals from diseased ones. Improved diagnostics are critical to TB care and control.

The need for serious investment in the critical areas especially in new TB diagnostic tools, drug susceptibility testing, and development of new biomarkers to enable health providers detect TB disease activity and to determine follow up treatment outcomes cannot be over emphasised. The fact that a number of new diagnostic tools are in the pipeline, including culture-based tests to identify M. tuberculosis and those used to determine drug resistance based on molecular assays and immune response is good news. However, there is still need to ensure that the new tests can be availed world-wide and be used at the point-of-care even in resource-poor settings, where there may be limited technical expertise and the necessary equipment. [http://ec.europa.eu/research/research-eu]

6.3. Newer biomarkers for TB disease activity, cure and relapse

There are three major reasons that can be used to justify the need for new TB biomarkers : 1) a diagnostic test which is able to differentiate between healthy individuals with a latent TB infection and patients with active dsease is needed; 2) a prognostic test which can be able to predict the risk of latent TB becoming active needs to be established; 3) there is need for a diagnostic test that can be used to serve as a surrogate endpoint of disease which can be used for monitoring drug and vaccine trials in TB. It is envisaged that the basis for these novel diagnostic measures will be biomics, comprising metabolomic, proteomic and transcriptomic profiles in custom-made biosignature. Identification of non invasive biomarkers, especially the molecular assay of M. tuberculosi fragments in urine and the measurement of volatile biomarkers of volatile organic compounds generated by Mycobacteria TB in the breath or the oxidative stress resulting from infection is one step in the right direction. [http://ec.europa.eu/research/research-eu]

6.4. Need for post-exposure vaccines and those effective against all M. tuberculosis strains

The Bacille Calmette-Guerin (BCG) vaccine is currently the only vaccine in use against tuberculosis. The efficacy of this vaccine is limited to prevention of severe forms of tuberculosis among children and there are lots of problems in cases of TB/ HIV coinfection.The current vaccine candidates are being developed for pre-exposure administration but, considering the fact that one third of the world's population is already infected, there is a serious need for a post-exposure vaccine to prevent re-activation. Another shortcoming with the vaccines in the pipeline is that they can delay clinical TB but cannot achieve sterile eradication. There is need for combination vaccines that can combine the effects of booster vaccines with another generation of vaccines that can act to effect sterilisation at the post-exposure stage. Focus should also be put on the development of a vaccine that can afford protection against the wide range of M. tuberculosis strains, to ensure universal effectiveness.To avoid complications in clinical and epidemiological research, the evaluation of all the vaccines should also deal with confounding factors such as prior BCG vaccination or HIV status and there should be well worked out guidelines for use of these vaccines in children [http//www.ec.europa.eu/research/research-eu]

6.5. Development of new drugs

When it comes to the current status of clinical, diagnostic and therapeutic strategies, childhood TB has been grossly neglected and there is, therefore need for better and standardized treatment strategy. Although there is a reasonable number of candidates in the discovery and pre-clinical pipeline, there are still gaps between the different stages of TB drug development, and drugs specically targeting paediatric TB are still needed. Most of the drugs in the pipeline use the same mechanisms with the majority aimed at boosting efficacy or shortening the duration, with very few targeingt dormant stages of the bacillus and, therefore, not suitable for eradication of latent infections. Thus urgency for serious research into the development of new drugs and treatment regimens aimed at achieving this therapeutic objective cannot be over emphasised. Dealing with TB/HIV co-infection is another gap that needs serious attention: there is need to develop drugs that can prevent dormant mycobacteria from re-activating in HIV-positive individuals [http://ec.europa.eu/research/research-eu.

7. Future prospects

7.1. Reducing the burden of childhood tuberculosis

TB in children presents a number of difficult challenges which will only be solved by a shift in research priorities. Advances in paediatric TB research will provide wider insights and opportunities for TB control. While development of a new vaccine to prevent TB should be the ultimate goal, development of better diagnostics represent one of the most important steps towards improving individual case management and also providing a more robust case definition for much needed drug and vaccine trials for studies on TB epidemiology and correlates of protective immunity in childhood. Data on the epidemiology of childhood TB may in turn help to inform public health policy by providing a window on current transmission and the effectiveness of control strategies and by identifying children with LTBI for chemo-prophylaxis to limit the future propagation of the epidemic. Emphasis should be placed on reducing the vulnerability of the community because successful control of the tuberculosis epidemic is the most effective way to reduce the burden of childhood tuberculosis However, this will require a holistic approach with sustainable poverty alleviation as a key element [http://www. ec.europa.eu/research/research-eu].

7.2. Involvement of funders and industry

Important resources are required for the exploration of pathways leading to TB diagnostics-oriented basic science in pathogen biology, biomarker discovery, systems biology and point of care test development. The current priorities for TB vaccine development are: i) new vaccine candidates that achieve sterile eradication, and that can progress into phase II and phase III trials; ii) vaccine testing in a naïve stage on M. tuberculosis uninfected individuals; iii) vaccines which can achieve post-exposure prophylaxis to those who are already infected (currently 2 billion people); iv) strategies on how to get vaccines from the research bench to the bedside and into the community. Apart from the protective effect of novel vaccine candidates, priority should be given also to their delivery route, formulation (storage, shelf-life and distribution) and utility for HIV-infected individuals, particularly children.

7.3. Back to basic research

As we talk about nano technology and pin point delivery of drugs it is a shame that 130 years after the Robert Koch's discovery of M. Tuberculosis we still have huge gaps in our under-standing of the biology, immunology and pathophysiology of the bacillus. We are, as yet, not able to explain fully the molecular, biochemical and immunological mechanisms that enable TB infection to go on for years and cause severe disease and death. With the availability of state-of-the-art molecular research tools such as functional genomics and metabolomics a paradigm shift towards empahsising basic research could help provide answers to some of the unanswered questions about M.tuberculosis in general, and paediatric TB in particular. The currently available knowledge has proved insufficient when it comes to the rational design of vaccines or other control tools and this has resulted in a lot of trial-and-error approaches. With the HIV virus still elusive, defeating the dual alliance of TB/HIV co-infection has added another diamension in the already complicated war against the resistant strains of M. tuberculosis. Promoting basic research by providing the necessary resources and involving stakehoolders on the political front can provide solutions to some of the outstanding problems if not solving all of them. Where there is will, there is a way [http//ec.europa.eu/research/research-eu].

7.4. Concluding remarks

Recent developments for TB diagnostics seem promising fields due to the fact they are fast and minimally invasive, but they have drawbacks of not being validated in diverse populations and improved according to the patient's needs. Refinement of existing tools and development and testing of new tools are urgently required to improve diagnosis and treatment of TB in children. Higher global priority and funding will be required to improve on childhood nutrition and promote improvement in the socioeconomic and environmental condition of communities if we are to have a significant impact on TB transmission to children. [Expand +Clinical Infectious Diseasescid.oxfordjournals.org

Author details

Claude Kirimuhuzya*

Address all correspondence to: claudekirim@yahoo.co.uk

Address all correspondence to: kirimuhuzya@gmail.com

Department of Pharmacology and Toxicology, Faculty of Biomedical Sciences, Kampala International University-Western Campus, Bushenyi, Uganda

References

[1] Nelson, L. J, & Wells, C. D. (2004). Global epidemiology of childhood tuberculosis. Int J Tuberc Lung Dis. , 8, 636-647.

[2] Nelson, L. J, Schneider, E, Wells, C. D, & Moore, M. (2004). Epidemiology of childhood tuberculosis in the United States, 1993-2001: the need for continued vigilance," Pediatrics, 114 (2 I): , 333-341.

[3] Donald, P. R, Schaaf, H. S, & Schoeman, J. F. (2005). Tuberculous meningitis and miliary tuberculosis: the Rich focus revisited. J Infect Dis. , 50, 193-195.

[4] Donald, P. R, Sirgel, F. A, Venter, A, Parkin, D. P, & Seifart, H. I. van de Wal BW, Werely C, van Helden PD, Maritz JS ((2004). The influence of human N-acetyltrans-

ferase genotype on the early bactericidal activity of isoniazid. Clin Infect Dis. , 39, 1425-1430.

[5]   Donald, P. R, & Schoeman, J. F. (2004). Tuberculous meningitis. N Engl J Med. 2004 Oct 21;, 351(17), 1719-20.

[6]   Starke, J. R. (2002). Childhood tuberculosis: ending the neglect. Int J Tuberc Lung Dis. , 6, 373-374.

[7]   Starke, J. R. (2003). Pediatric tuberculosis: time for a new approach. Tuberculosis (Edinb). , 83, 208-212.

[8]   Marais, B. J, Hesseling, A. C, Gie, R. P, Schaaf, H. S, & Beyers, N. (2006). The burden of childhood tuberculosis and the accuracy of routine surveillance data in a high-burden setting. Int J Tuberc Lung Dis. , 10, 259-263.

[9]   Marais, B. J, Gie, R. P, Schaaf, H. S, Hesseling, A. C, Obihara, C. C, Starke, J. J, Enarson, D. A, Donald, P. R, & Beyers, N. (2004). The natural history of disease of childhood intra-thoracic tuberculosis: a critical review of the prechemotherapy literature. Int J Tuberc Lung Dis. , 8, 392-402.

[10] Marais, B. J, Obihara, C. C, Gie, R. P, Schaaf, H. S, Hesseling, A. C, Lombard, C, Enarson, D, Bateman, E, & Beyers, N. (2005). The prevalence of symptoms associated with pulmonary tuberculosis in randomly selected children from a high-burden community. Arch Dis Child. , 90, 1166-1170.

[11] Marais, B. J, & Pai, M. (2007). Recent advances in the diagnosis of childhood tuberculosis. Arch Dis Child. , 92(5), 446-52.

[12] Schaaf, H. S, Marais, B. J, Hesseling, A. C, Brittle, W, & Donald, P. R. (2009). Surveillance of antituberculosis drug resistance among children from the Western Cape Province of South Africa-an upward trend. Am J Public Health. , 99, 1486-1490.

[13] Schaaf, H. S, Parkin, D. P, Seifart, H. I, et al. (2005). Jun Isoniazid pharmacokinetics in children treated for respiratory tuberculosis. Arch Dis Child. , 90(6), 614-8.

[14] Schaaf, H. S, Cotton, M. F, & Zar, H. J. (2007). Failure of chemoprophylaxis with standard antituberculosis agents in child contacts of multidrug-resistant tuberculosis cases. Pediatr Infect Dis J 2007;, 26, 1142-1146.

[15] Hesseling, A. C, Cotton, M. F, Marais, B. J, et al. (2007). BCG and HIV reconsidered: moving the research agenda forward. Vaccine. , 25(36), 6565-8.

[16] Hesseling, A. C, Rabie, H, Marais, B. J, Manders, M, Lips, M, Schaaf, H. S, Warren, R. M, Gie, R. P, Cotton, M. F, Van Helden, P, et al. (2006). Bacille Calmette-Guerin (BCG) vaccine-induced complications and HIV infection in children. Clin Infect Dis. , 42, 548-558.

[17] Hesseling, A. C, Schaaf, H. S, Gie, R. P, Starke, J. R, & Beyers, N. (2002). A critical review of diagnostic approaches used in the diagnosis of childhood tuberculosis. Int J Tuberc Lung Dis. , 6, 1038-1045.

[18] Walters, E, Cotton, M. F, Rabie, H, Schaaf, H. S, Walters, L. O, & Marais, B. J. (2006). Clinical presentation and outcome of Tuberculosis in Human Immunodeficiency Virus infected children on anti-retroviral therapy. BMC Pediatr. 8(1):1.

[19] Van Zyl, S, Marais, B. J, Hesseling, A. C, Gie, R. P, Beyers, N, & Schaaf, H. S. (2006). Adherence to antituberculosis chemoprophylaxis and treatment in children. Int J Tuberc Lung Dis. , 10, 13-18.

[20] Brittle, W, Marais, B. J, Hesseling, A. C, et al. (2009). Improvement in mycobacterial yield and reduced time to detection in pediatric samples by use of a nutrient broth growth supplement. J Clin Microbiol. , 47, 1287-1289.

[21] Chintu, C, Mudenda, V, Lucas, S, et al. (2002). Lung diseases at necropsy in African children dying from respiratory illnesses: a descriptive necropsy study. Lancet. , 360(9338), 985-90.

[22] Andronikou, S, Joseph, E, Lucas, S, & Brachmeyer, S. Du Toit G, Zar H, Swingler G ((2004). CT scanning for the detection of tuberculous mediastinal and hilar lymphadenopathy in children. Pediatr Radiol; , 34, 232-236.

[23] Verver, S, Warren, R. M, Munch, Z, Richardson, M, Van Der Spuy, G. D, Borgdorff, M. W, Behr, M. A, Beyers, N, & Van Helden, P. D. (2004). Proportion of tuberculosis transmission that takes place in households in a high-incidence area. Lancet. , 363, 212-214.

[24] Van den BoschTerken M, Ypma L, Kimpen JL, Nel ED, Schaaf HS, Schoeman JF, Donald PR ((2004). Tuberculous meningitis and miliary tuberculosis in young children. Trop Med Int Health; , 9, 309-313.

[25] Zar, H. J, Hanslo, D, Apolles, P, Swingler, G, & Hussey, G. (2005). Induced sputum versus gastric lavage for microbiological confirmation confirmation of pulmonary tuberculosis in infants and young children: a prospective study. Lancet; , 365, 130-134.

[26] Zar, H, Cotton, M. F, Strauss, S, et al. (2007). Effect of isoniazid prophylaxis on mortality and incidence of tuberculosis in children with HIV: a randomized clinical trial. BMJ. , 334, 105-106.

[27] American Thoracic Society ((2000). Targeted tuberculin testing and treatment of latent tuberculosis infection. Am J Respir Crit Care Med. 161:SS247., 221.

[28] Graham, S. M. Coulter JBS, Gilks CF, ((2001). Pulmonary disease in HIV-infected children. Int J Tuberc Lung Dis. , 5, 12-23.

[29] Graham, S. M, Gie, R. P, Schaaf, H. S, Coulter, J. B. S, Espinal, M. A, & Beyers, N. (2004). Childhood tuberculosis: clinical research needs," International Journal of Tuberculosis and Lung Disease, 8(5): 648-657,

[30] Chow, F, Espiritu, N, Gilman, R. H, et al. (2006). La cuerda dulce--a tolerability and acceptability study of a novel approach to specimen collection for diagnosis of paediatric pulmonary tuberculosis. BMC Infect Dis. 6:67.

[31] Moore, D. A, Evans, C. A, Gilman, R. H, et al. (2006). Microscopic-observation drug-susceptibility assay for the diagnosis of TB. N Engl J Med. 12;, 355(15), 1539-50.

[32] Sarmiento, O. L, Weigle, K. A, Alexander, J, Weber, D. J, & Miller, W. C. (2003). Assessment by meta-analysis of PCR for diagnosis of smear-negative pulmonary tuberculosis. J Clin Microbiol. , 41(7), 3233-40.

[33] Kocagoz, T, Brien, O, & Perkins, R. M ((2004). A new colorimetric culture system for the diagnosis of tuberculosis. Int J Tuberc Lung Dis. 8(12):1512.

[34] Fend, R, Kolk, A. H, Bessant, C, Buijtels, P, Klatser, P. R, & Woodman, A. C. (2006). Prospects for clinical application of electronic-nose technology to early detection of Mycobacterium tuberculosis in culture and sputum. J Clin Microbiol. , 44(6), 2039-45.

[35] Oberhelman, R. A, Soto-castellares, G, Caviedes, L, et al. (2006). Improved recovery of Mycobacterium tuberculosis from children using the microscopic observation drug susceptibility method. Pediatrics. 118(1):e, 100-6.

[36] Arend, S. M, Thijsen, S. F, Leyten, E. M, et al. (2007). Comparison of two interferon-gamma assays and tuberculin skin test for tracing tuberculosis contacts. Am J Respir Crit Care Med. 15;, 175(6), 618-27.

[37] Clark, S. A, Martin, S. L, Pozniak, A, et al. (2007). Tuberculosis antigen-specific immune responses can be detected using enzyme-linked immunospot technology in human immunodeficiency virus (HIV)-1 patients with advanced disease. Clin Exp Immunol. , 150(2), 238-44.

[38] Steingart, K. R, Henry, M, Laal, S, et al. (2007). A systematic review of commercial serological antibody detection tests for the diagnosis of extrapulmonary tuberculosis. Thorax. , 62(10), 911-8.

[39] WHO ((2006). The Global Plan to Stop TB, Annex 1 Methods used to estimate costs, funding and funding gaps..., 2006-2015.

[40] World Health Organization (WHO) ((2007). Stop TB Partnership Childhood TB Subgroup. Childhood Contact screening and management. Int J Tuberc Lung Dis. , 11(1), 12-5.

[41] World Health Organization ((2003). Treatment of tuberculosis: guidelines for national programmes. 3rd ed. Geneva, Switzerland: World Health Organization.

[42] WHO Report ((2009). Global tuberculosis control-epidemiology, strategy, financing.

[43]   World Health Organization ((2010). WHO publications on tuberculosis.

[44]   World Health Organization ((2004). Guidelines for the management of drug-resistant tuberculosis. Geneva, Switzerland: World Health Organization.

[45]   Wells, C. D, Cegielski, J. P, Nelson, L. J, et al. (2007). HIV infection and multidrug-resistant tuberculosis: the perfect storm. J Infect Dis. 196 (Suppl 1):S, 86-107.

[46]   Soeters, M, De Vries, A. M, Kimpen, J. L, Donald, P. R, & Schaaf, H. S. (2005). Clinical features and outcome in children admitted to a TB hospital in the Western Cape--the influence of HIV infection and drug resistance. S Afr Med J. , 95(8), 602-6.

[47]   Roth, A, Garly, M. L, Jensen, H, Nielsen, J, & Aaby, P. (2006). Bacille Calmette-Guerin vaccination and infant mortality. Expert Rev Vaccines. , 5(2), 277-93.

[48]   Doherty, T. M, Dietrich, J, & Billeskov, R. (2007). Tuberculosis subunit vaccines: from basic science to clinical testing. Expert Opin Biol Ther. , 7(10), 1539-49.

[49]   Andersen, P. (2007). Vaccine strategies against latent tuberculosis infection. Trends Microbiol. , 15(1), 7-13.

[50]   Walls, T, & Shingadia, D. (2004). Global epidemiology of paediatric tuberculosis. J Infect. , 4813-22.

[51]   Corbett, E L, Watt, C J, Walker, N, et al. (2003). The growing burden of tuberculosis: global trends and interactions with the HIV epidemic. Arch Intern Med. , 1631009-1021.

[52]   Boehme, C, Molokova, E, Minja, F, et al. (2005). Detection of mycobacterial lipoarabinomannan with an antigen-capture ELISA in unprocessed urine of Tanzanian patients with suspected tuberculosis. Trans R Soc Trop Med Hyg. , 99893-900.

[53]   Pai, M, Gokhale, K, Joshi, R, et al. (2005). Mycobacterium tuberculosis infection in health care workers in rural India: comparison of a whole blood, interferon-® assay with tuberculin skin testing. JAMA. , 2932746-2755.

[54]   Pai, M, Kalantri, S, & Dheda, K. (2006). New tools and emerging technologies for the diagnosis of tuberculosis: Part 1. Latent tuberculosis. Expert Rev Mol Diag. , 6413-422.

[55]   Hill, P C, Brookes, R H, Adetifa, I, et al. (2006). Comparison of enzyme linked immunospot assay and tuberculin skin test in healthy children exposed to mycobacterium tuberculosis. Pediatrics , 1171542-1548.

[56]   Kalantri, S, Pai, M, Pascopella, L, et al. (2005). Bacteriophage-based tests for the detection of Mycobacterium tuberculosis in clinical specimens: a systematic review and meta-analysis. BMC Infect Dis. 559.

[57]   Dalton, T, Cegielski, P, Akksilp, S, Asencios, L, Caoili, J C, Cho, S-N, Erokhin, V. V, Ershova, J, Gler, T, Kazennyy, B Y, Kim, H J, Kliiman, K, Kurbatova, E, Kvasnovsky, C, Leimane, V, Van Der Walt, M P, Via, L E, Volchenkov, G. V, Yagui, M A, & Kang,

H. the Global PETTS ((2012). Prevalence of and risk factors for resistance to second-line drugs in people with multidrug-resistant tuberculosis in eight countries: a prospective cohort study. The Lancet, Early Online Publication, 30 August 2012

[58] Ferrara, G, Losi, M, Amico, D, Roversi, R, Piro, P, Meacci, R, Meccugni, M, Dori, B, Andreani, I. M, Bergamini, A, Mussini, B. M, Rumpianesi, C, Fabbri, F, & Richeldi, L. M. L ((2006). Use in routine clinical practice of two commercial blood tests for diagnosis of infection with Mycobacterium tuberculosis: a prospective study. Lancet. 22; , 367(9519), 1328-34.

[59] Salgado, E, & Gomez-reino, J. J. (2011). The risk of tuberculosis in patients treated with TNF antagonists. Expert Rev Clin Immunol. , 7(3), 329-40.

[60] Solovic, I, Sester, M, Gomez-reino, J. J, Rieder, H. L, Ehlers, S, Milburn, H. J, et al. (2010). The risk of tuberculosis related to tumour necrosis factor antagonist therapies: a TBNET consensus statement. Eur Respir J. 2010 Nov;, 36(5), 1185-206.

[61] Gomez-pastrana, D, Torronteras, R, Caro, P, et al. (2001). Comparison of amplicor, in-house polymerase chain reaction, and conventional culture for the diagnosis of tuberculosis in children," Clinical Infectious Diseases, , 32(1), 17-22.

[62] Montenegro, S. H, Gilman, R. H, Sheen, P, Cama, R, Caviedes, L, Hopper, T, Chambers, R, & Oberhelman, R. A. (2003). Improved detection of Mycobacterium tuberculosis in Peruvian children by use of a heminested IS6110 polymerase chain reaction assay. Clin Infect Dis. , 36, 16-23.

[63] Pai, M. (2004). The accuracy and reliability of nucleic acid amplification tests in the diagnosis of tuberculosis. Natl Med J India. , 17233-236.

[64] Mitchison, D. A. (2005). The diagnosis and therapy of tuberculosis during the past 100 years. Am J Respir Crit Care Med. , 171, 699-706.

[65] Blumberg, H. M, Burman, W. J, Chaisson, R. E, Daley, C. L, Etkind, S. C, Friedman, L. N, Fujiwara, P, Grzemska, M, Hopewell, P. C, Iseman, M. D, et al. (2003). American Thoracic Society, Centers for Disease Control and Prevention, Infectious Diseases Society. Treatment of tuberculosis. Am J Respir Crit Care Med. , 167, 603-662.

[66] European Centre for Disease Prevention and Control (ECDC) ((2012). Management of contacts of MDR TB and XDR TB patients. Stockholm: ECDC; 2012. Stockholm, March 2012 978-9-29193-336-5doi

[67] Dekker, T. G, & Lotter, A. P. (2003). Anti-tuberculosis 4FDC tablets: mystery to chemistry. Int J Tuberc Lung Dis. , 7, 205-206.

[68] Ena, J, & Valls, V. (2005). Short-course therapy with rifampin plus isoniazid, compared with standard therapy with isoniazid, for latent tuberculosis infection: a meta-analysis. Clin Infect Dis. , 40, 670-676.

[69] Priest, D. H, Vossel, L. F, Sherfy, E. A, Hoy, D. P, & Haley, C. A. (2004). Use of intermittent rifampin and pyrazinamide therapy for tuberculosis infection in a targeted tuberculin-testing program. Clin Infect Dis. , 15, 1764-1771.

[70] Al-dossary, F. S, Ong, L. T, Correa, A. G, & Starke, J. R. (2002). Treatment of childhood tuberculosis with a six month directly observed regimen of only two weeks of daily therapy. Pediatr Infect Dis J;, 21, 91-97.

[71] Bjarveit, K, Scheel, O, & Heimbeck, J. (2003). Their contribution to understanding the pathogenesis and prevention of tuberculosis. Int J Tuberc Lung Dis., 7, 306-311.

[72] American Academy of Pediatrics ((2003). Tuberculosis. In: Pickering LK, editor. Red book: report of the Committee on Infectious Diseases, 26th ed. Elk Grove Village, IL: Amercian Academy of Pediatrics , 650-651.

[73] Centers for Disease Control and Prevention (CDC)(2010). Mantoux tuberculosis skin test facilitator guide. Part two: reading the Mantoux tuberculin skin test.

[74] Rieder, H. L, Arnadottir, A, Trebucq, A, & Enarson, D. A. (2001). Tuberculosis treatment: dangerous regimens? Int J Tuberc Lung Dis. , 5, 1-3.

[75] Rieder, H. (2005). Annual risk of infection with Mycobacterium tuberculosis. Eur Respir J. , 25(1), 181-5.

[76] Newton, S. M, Smith, R. J, Wilkinson, K. A, et al. (2006). A deletion defining a common Asian lineage of Mycobacterium tuberculosis associates with immune subversion. Proc Natl Acad Sci U S A. , 103(42), 15594-8.

[77] Newton, S. M, Brent, A. J, Anderson, S, Whittaker, E, & Kampmann, B. (2008). Paedatric Tuberculosis. Lancet Infect Dis., 8(8), 498-510.

[78] Lalvani, A, & Millington, K. A. diagnosis of childhood tuberculosis infection. Curr Opin Infect Dis. , 20, 264-271.

[79] López Ávalos GG and Montes de Oca E P ((2012). Review Article Classic and New Diagnostic Approaches to Childhood Tuberculosis. Journal of Tropical Medicine Article ID 818219, 12 pages, 2012

[80] Nicol, M. P, & Zar, H. J. (2011). New specimens and laboratory diagnostics for childhood pulmonary TB: progress and prospects," Paediatric Respiratory Reviews., 12(1), 16-21.

[81] Nicol, M. P, Davies, M. A, Wood, K, et al. (2009). Comparison of T-SPOT. TB assay and tuberculin skin test for the evaluation of young children at high risk for tuberculosis in a community setting," Pediatrics. , 123(1), 38-43.

[82] Nicol, M. P, Workman, L, Isaacs, W, et al. (2011). Accuracy of the Xpert MTB/RIF test for the diagnosis of pulmonary tuberculosis in children admitted to hospital in Cape Town, South Africa: a descriptive study," The Lancet Infectious Diseases, , 11(11), 819-824.

[83] Dogra, S, Narang, P, Mendiratta, D. K, et al. (2007). Comparison of a whole blood in-terferon-γ assay with tuberculin skin testing for the detection of tuberculosis infection in hospitalized children in rural India," Journal of Infection. , 54(3), 267-276.

[84] Edwards, D. J. Kitetele, and Van Rie A., ((2007). Agreement between clinical scoring systems used F. for the diagnosis of pediatric tuberculosis in the HIV era," International Journal of Tuberculosis and Lung Disease., 11(3), 263-269.

[85] Lewinsohn, D. A, Gennaro, M. L, Scholvinck, L, & Lewinsohn, D. M. (2004). Tuberculosis immunology in children: diagnostic and therapeutic challenges and opportunities," International Journal of Tuberculosis and Lung Disease. , 8(5), 658-674.

[86] Imaz, M. S, Comini, M. A, Zerbini, E, et al. (2001). Evaluation of the diagnostic value of measuring IgG, IgM and IgA antibodies to the recombinant 16-kilodalton antigen of Mycobacterium tuberculosis in childhood tuberculosis," International Journal of Tuberculosis and Lung Disease. , 5(11), 1036-1043.

[87] Detjen, A. K, Keil, T, Roll, S, et al. (2007). Interferon-γamma release assays improve the diagnosis of tuberculosis and non-tuberculous mycobacterial disease in children in a country with a low incidence of tuberculosis. Clin Infect Dis. , 45, 322-328.

[88] Bakir, M, Millington, K. A, Soysal, A, et al. (2008). Prognostic value of a T-cell-based, interferon-γ biomarker in children with tuberculosis contact," Annals of Internal Medicine. , 149(11), 777-786.

[89] Dinnes, J, Deeks, J, Kunst, H, et al. (2007). A systematic review of rapid diagnostic tests for the detection of tuberculosis infection," Health Technology Assessment, , 11(3), 1-196.

[90] Rachow, A, Zumla, A, Heinrich, N, et al. (2011). Rapid and accurate detection of Mycobacterium tuberculosis in sputum samples by Cepheid Xpert MTB/RIF assay-a clinical validation study," PLoS ONE, article e20458,., 6(6)

[91] Liang, Q. L, Shi, H. Z, Wang, K, Qin, S. M, & Qin, X. J. (2008). Diagnostic accuracy of adenosine deaminase in tuberculous pleurisy: a meta-analysis," Respiratory Medicine. , 102(5), 744-754.

[92] Lawn, S. D, & Nicol, M. P. (2011). Xpert MTB/RIF assay: development, evaluation and implementation of a new rapid molecular diagnostic for tuberculosis and rifampicin resistance," Future Microbiology,. , 6(9), 1067-1082.

[93] Trilling, A. K, De Ronde, H, Noteboom, L, et al. (2011). A broad set of different llama antibodies specific for a 16 kda heat shock protein of mycobacterium tuberculosis," PLoS ONE, article e26754, 6(10)

[94] Gordetsov, A. S, Mamaeva, L. A, Krylov, V. N, & Lebedev, A. V. (2008). Method of respiratory active tuberculosis diagnostics," RU2327990 (C1), Russia.

[95] Swaminathan, S, & Rekha, B. (2010). Pediatric Tuberculosis: Global Overview and Challenges. Clin Infect Dis. 50 (Supplement 3

[96] Jeena, P. M, Pillay, P, Pillay, T, & Coovadia, H. M. (2002). Impact of HIV-1 co-infection on presentation and hospital-related mortality in children with culture proven pulmonary tuberculosis in Durban, South Africa. Int J Tuberc Lung Dis. , 6(8), 672-8.

[97] Rekha, B, & Swaminathan, S. (2007). Childhood tuberculosis-global epidemiology and the impact of HIV. Pediatr Respir Rev , 8, 99-106.

[98] Drobac, P. C, Mukherjee, J. S, Joseph, J. K, et al. (2006). Community-based therapy for children with multidrug-resistant tuberculosis. Pediatrics. , 117(6), 2022-9.

[99] AAP(1996). Update on tuberculosis skin testing of children. American Academy of Pediatrics Committee on Infectious Diseases. Pediatrics. , 97(2), 282-4.

[100] Saiman, L. San Gabriel P, Schulte J, Vargas MP, Kenyon T, Onorato I ((2001). Risk factors for latent tuberculosis infection among children in New York City. Pediatrics. , 107(5), 999-1003.

[101] Shingadia, D, & Novelli, V. (2003). Diagnosis and treatment of tuberculosis in children. Lancet Infect Dis. , 3(10), 624-32.

[102] Cegielski, J. P, & Mcmurray, D. N. (2004). The relationship between malnutrition and tuberculosis: evidence from studies in humans and experimental animals. Int J Tuberc Lung Dis. 2004 Mar;, 8(3), 286-98.

[103] Palme, I. B, Gudetta, B, Bruchfeld, J, Muhe, L, & Giesecke, J. (2002). Impact of human immunodeficiency virus 1 infection on clinical presentation, treatment outcome and survival in a cohort of Ethiopian children with tuberculosis. Pediatr Infect Dis J. , 21(11), 1053-61.

[104] Brent, A. J, Anderson, S. T, & Kampmann, B. (2007). Childhood tuberculosis: out of sight, out of mind? Trans R Soc Trop Med Hyg.

[105] Bryce, J, Boschi-pinto, C, Shibuya, K, & Black, R. E. (2005). WHO estimates of the causes of death in children. Lancet. , 365(9465), 1147-52.

[106] Scott, J. A, Brooks, W. A, Peiris, J. S, Holtzman, D, & Mulhollan, E. K. (2008). Pneumonia research to reduce childhood mortality in the developing world. J Clin Invest. , 118(4), 1291-300.

[107] Upham, J. W, Lee, P. T, Holt, B. J, et al. (2002). Development of interleukin-12-producing capacity throughout childhood. Infect Immun. , 70(12), 6583-8.

[108] Kampmann, B, Hemingway, C, Stephens, A, et al. (2005). Acquired predisposition to mycobacterial disease due to autoantibodies to IFN-gamma. J Clin Invest. , 115(9), 2480-8.

[109]   Kampmann, B, Tena-coki, G. N, Nicol, M. P, Levin, M, & Eley, B. (2006). Reconstitu-
        tion of antimycobacterial immune responses in HIV-infected children receiving
        HAART. Aids. , 20(7), 1011-8.

[110]   Van Der Weert, E. M, Hartgers, N. M, Schaaf, H. S, et al. (2006). Comparison of diag-
        nostic criteria of tuberculous meningitis in human immunodeficiency virus-infected
        and uninfected children. Pediatr Infect Dis J. , 25(1), 65-9.

[111]   Meya, D. B, & Mcadam, K. P. (2007). The TB pandemic: an old problem seeking new
        solutions. J Intern Med. , 261(4), 309-29.

[112]   Tena, G. N, Young, D. B, Eley, B, et al. (2003). Failure to control growth of mycobacte-
        ria in blood from children infected with human immunodeficiency virus and its rela-
        tionship to T cell function. J Infect Dis. , 187(10), 1544-51.

[113]   Elenga, N, Kouakoussui, K. A, Bonard, D, et al. (2005). Diagnosed tuberculosis dur-
        ing the follow-up of a cohort of human immunodeficiency virus-infected children in
        Abidjan, Cote d'Ivoire: ANRS 1278 study. Pediatr Infect Dis J. , 24(12), 1077-82.

[114]   Anderson, S. T, Williams, A. J, Brown, J. R, et al. (2006). Transmission of Mycobacteri-
        um tuberculosis undetected by tuberculin skin testing. Am J Respir Crit Care Med.,
        173(9), 1038-42.

[115]   Thwaites, G. E, & Tran, T. H. (2005). Tuberculous meningitis: many questions, too
        few answers. Lancet Neurol. , 4(3), 160-70.

[116]   Rodrigues, L. C, Pereira, S. M, Cunha, S. S, et al. (2005). Effect of BCG revaccination
        on incidence of tuberculosis in school-aged children in Brazil: the BCG-REVAC clus-
        ter-randomised trial. Lancet. , 366(9493), 1290-5.

[117]   Chen, Z. W. (2004). Immunology of AIDS virus and mycobacterial co-infection. Curr
        HIV Res. , 2(4), 351-5.

[118]   [http://wwwec.europa.eu/research/research-eu] accessed on August 1st (2012).

[119]   Shah(2012). Espid Reports And Reviews at: www.pidj.com].Accessed on18th August
        2012

Chapter 4

Research and Development of New Drugs Against Tuberculosis

Juan D. Guzman, Ximena Montes-Rincón and
Wellman Ribón

Additional information is available at the end of the chapter

1. Introduction

Tuberculosis (TB) is a contagious infectious disease caused by species belonging to the *Mycobacterium tuberculosis* complex. At present, it is a re-emerging disease, due to co-infection with the Human Immunodeficiency Virus (HIV), but also to global bacterial resistance, and lack of adequate treatment in some places in the world. Approximately one third of the world's population is infected with *M. tuberculosis*, and out of these people, about 1.1 million people die every year of TB [1], making this disease the main cause of bacterial infectious death in adolescents and adults all around the world. In 2010 there was an estimation of 8.8 million incident cases and 12.0 million prevalent cases of TB worldwide. *M. tuberculosis* drug-resistant isolates have appeared giving origin to multidrug-resistant (MDR) and extensively drug-resistant (XDR) strains. XDR-TB has been identified in every continent of the planet. By 2010, the World Health Organization (WHO) was notified of the existence of 53.018 cases of multi-drug resistant TB (MDR-TB) worldwide; figure that only represents 18% of the TB-MDR estimated cases among reported pulmonary TB cases around the world [1]. Currently, there is global alarm since the infection with these strains is cured only in 66% of MDR cases and in 60% of the XDR cases [2].

More than sixty years ago, the introduction of the first anti-TB drugs for the treatment of TB (streptomycin (STR), *p*-aminosalcylic acid (PAS), isoniazid (INH) and then later ethambutol (EMB) and rifampicin (RIF)) gave optimism to the medical community, and it was believed that the disease would be completely eradicated soon. After a 30-year halt of anti-TB drug Research & Development pipeline, the Global Alliance for TB Drug Development (TB Alliance) started to fill the gap between the existing chemotherapeutics and the clinical need. Despite the efforts carried out with candidates in clinical trials such as PA-824 and bedaquiline, there is an urgent need of in-depth medicinal chemistry discovery studies for assuring enough leads and candidates feeding the pipeline within the next decade[3]. Emerging chemical entities must shorten the time of treatment, be potent and safe while effective facing resistant strains and non-replicative, latent forms, and not interfere in the antiretroviral therapy [4]. In this review, we explore why we require to work continuously on the development of novel anti-TB agents, the stages necessary for the development of new anti-TB agents, breakthroughs in the discovery of new active principles and targets, the preclinical and clinical development of drugs, as well as the new approaches for the search of anti-TB active principles.

2. Targets and action mode of active principles currently used in the treatment of TB

Current TB chemotherapy is based on the combination of four anti-TB drugs which inhibit the bacterial metabolism, particularly the cell wall synthesis [5]. During the therapy, the goal of this drug combination strategy is to prevent effectively the mutational events [6]. According to their action mode, first and second line anti-TB drugs are grouped into cell wall inhibitors (INH, EMB, ethionamide (ETH), and cycloserine (DCS)), protein synthesis inhibitors (RIF, fluoroquinolones, STR, kanamycin (KAN)), and membrane energy metabolism inhibitors (PZA).

Current chemotherapy principally inhibits cell processes such as cell wall biosynthesis and DNA replication, and they only turn to be active regarding bacteria in active growth [5]. This implies that the chemotherapeutic agents in use are efficient bactericides but are poor sterilizers, not able to kill "dormant" M. tuberculosis which persists in macrophages after the death of the active bacteria [5]. RIF and PZA have a partial sterilizing activity and they play an important role in the decrease of therapy from 18 to 6 months, even though there is a persistent population surviving these two agents. Consequently the current therapy ensures a clinical cure but fails to obtain a bacteriological cure [5].

3. Why we need new active anti-TB agents?

Whereas it is true that TB can be cured with the current active principles, treatment is complex and long, involving four drugs for two months and two drugs for four months more as a minimum.

Active principle (year of discovery)	Source	MIC (µM)	Action mechanism	Target site	Genes involved in the resistance
First Line — Isoniazid (1952)	Synthetic	0.182	Mycolic acids synthesis inhibition, multiple effects on DNA, lipids and carbohydrates	Enoylreductase (InhA)	katG, inhA, ndh

Active principle (year of discovery)	Source	MIC (µM)	Action mechanism	Target site	Genes involved in the resistance
Rifampicin (1966)	Semi-synthetic	0.486	RNA synthesis inhibition	RNA polymerase β sub-unit	rpoB
Pyrazinamide (1952)	Synthetic	490 pH 5.5	Breakage of transport membrane and energetic depletion	Membrane energy metabolism	pncA
Ethambutol (1961)	Synthetic	2.45	Aarabinogalactanbiosynthesisinhibition	Arabinosyltransferase	embCAB
Streptomycin (1944)	Natural	1.72	Protein synthesis inhibition	rRNA ribosomal proteins S12 and 16S	rpsL, rrs
Kanamycin (1957)	Natural	3.43	Protein synthesis inhibition	rRNA ribosomal proteins S12 and 16S	rpsL, rrs
Amikacin (1972)	Semi-synthetic	0.85-1.7	Protein synthesis inhibition	rRNA ribosomal proteins S12 and 16S	rpsL, rrs
Fluoroquinolones (1980s)	Synthetic	0.6-1.4	DNA replication and transcription inhibition	DNA gyrase	gyrA, gyrB
Ethionamide (1956)	Synthetic	1.5	Mycolic acid biosynthesis inhibition	Enoylreductase (InhA)	inhA, etaA/ethA
Prothionamide	Synthetic	2.77	Mycolic acid biosynthesis inhibition	Enoylreductase (InhA)	inhA, etaA/ethA
p-aminosalicilic acid (1946)	Synthetic	1.9-6.5	Inhibition of thymidilate synthase and iron acquisition	Thymidilate synthase	thyA
Cycloserine (1952)	Natural	245	Peptidoglycan synthesis inhibition	D-alanine racemase	alrA,ddl

Second Line (marked at left side for Ethionamide through Cycloserine rows)

Table 1. Reported MIC and molecular targets drugs of first and second-line drugs used in the treatment of TB [7].

Since the start of chemotherapeutic era, physicians have realized the slowness and difficulty of achieving effective cure. McDermott et al proved in 1956 that the *in vitro*efficacy of first-line TB drugsdo not correlate to their *in vivo* efficacy [5]. Cultures of *M. tuberculosis* in exponential growth are sterilized *in vitro* in a few days by firstline agents such as INH and RIF, while the same combination requires months to achieve the same result in host tissue. It has been stated that mycobacterial persistency is due to the physiologic heterogeneity of bacillus in the tissues, the existence of subpopulations with completely different rate-determining factors. Despite an urgent need for new therapies targeting persistent bacteria, our knowledge of bacterial metabolism throughout the course of infection remains rudimentary [8].Mitchison and colleagues proposed in 1979 that, in lesions, *M. tuberculosis*exists under at least four different population stages listed below [9] and showed in Figure 1:

1. Bacteria in active growth, susceptible to INH.

2. Bacteria with intermittent metabolism period, susceptible to RIF.

3. Low metabolic activity bacteria residing in acidic pH, susceptible to PZA.

4. "Dormant" or "persistent" bacteria, non susceptible to any current active principle.

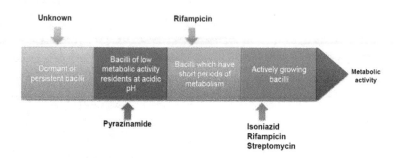

Figure 1. Spectrum of *M. tuberculosis*physiology.Extent of variation of physiological cell subpopulations of *M. tuberculosis* on an *in vivo* environment. Notice that first-line drugs mainly inhibit actively dividing bacteria, while there is not a single agent targeting the lower physiologically active stages.

During the initial chemotherapy phase (2 months), actively dividing bacilli rapidly die mostly because of INH bactericidal activity. Thereafter bacilli of low metabolic activity suffer from a slow death under the effects of RIF and PZA. There is evidence that persistentbacillarpopulation existing in the lesions usually determines the duration oftherapy [9]. Therefore efforts need to be made to target every physiological state of *M. tuberculosis* thus shortening the time of therapy and the appearance of drug resistance.

That brings us to the second reason why we need new anti-TB drugs. Drug resistance has emerged as a phantom from the dark, threatening today every corner of the world. RIF-resistance often correlates to MDR category (resistant to INH and RIF). XDR *M. tuberculosis* is an MDR strain also resistant to any fluoroquinolone and at least one injectable agent. Prognosis is less favorable for patients harboring XDR-bacilly compared to patients with MDR, with five times higher risk of death, require longer hospitalization or treatment times. However it has been shown that within an aggressive treatment, XDR-TB patients have been successfully cured in 60% [10,11]. Treatment of M/XDR-TB usually takes more than two years, and requires the use of more toxic, less effective and more expensive drugs. In resource-limiting countries, supplies of second-line drugs cannot be guaranteed. In an attempt to improve the conditions for millions of patients, Jim Yong Kim and Paul Farmer from Partners in Health brought down the price of second-line drugs has by more than 80%. Unfortunately the latest reports from Italy, India and Iran, facing the extremely (XXDR) or totally (TDR) super-bug, have made imperious the essential necessity of new drugs targeting novel mechanisms of action [12].

TB infection in immune-compromisedpopulation leads tosevere cases,possibly affecting other parts of the body, such as the pleura, meninges, the lymphatic system, the genitourinary system, and the bones [13]. It has been estimated that HIV infected patients are 100 times more likely to develop TB [14]. Although the studies support a decrease of mortality for TB patients after the introduction of antiretroviral therapy, evidence of the existence of interactions between Highly active antiretroviral therapy (HAART)and TB chemotherapy. HAAR is based on a combination therapynormally involving two reverse-transcriptase inhibitors and a non-inhibitor [15]. P450 Cytochrometypicallymetabolizes reverse-transcriptase inhibitors,however this cytochrome is also induced by RIF. TB chemotherapy may reduce significantly the concentrations of anti-retroviral drugs which may lead to treatment failure or resistance. An increase of the nevirapine dose to compensate for this interaction increases the risk of toxic effects and hepatotoxicity in patients who already present a low body mass index and high level of CD4 lymphocytes [16]. Physicians prefer to avoid the concomitant use of nevirapine and RIF; consequently there is a clinical need for mycobactericidal agents devoid of P450 catabolism.

4. A 50-year wait

Antibiotic discovery began in the early 1930s when different classes were discovered [17]. At the end of the 1950 decade, the combined regime was established and was thought to eradicate the disease completely. In the following thirty years after the introduction of the last first-line anti-TB drug, RIF, the regimen remained unchanged. The landscape changed in 1993 when the WHO declared TB a global health emergency [18]. Until recently, research in development of new anti-TB drugs was poor. These days, the TB Alliance has emerged as a non-profit organization promoting and funding anti-TB drug development by creating consortia over a defined project involving oftenbig pharmacompanies, institutes of research, and universities. Interest in drug discovery has placed on both phenotypic and target-based approaches to set in motion strong pipeline. With the joint effort of the Working Group on New TB Drugs, Stop TB Partnership and other societies.gatifloxacin, delamanib, PA824, rifapentine, sutezolid, SQ-109, bedaquiline and linezolid are candidatesin clinical trial [19]. There are other promising compounds (CPZEN-45, BTZ043, AZD5847, DC-159a and others), but a handful ofscientists believe that the gap is large and there is no certainty whether there will be a full new regimen in the next decade [3].

Neglected diseases affect mostly the poorest population on Earth, predominantly those who live in remote, rural areas, in depressed urban settings, or in regions of conflict. Together with malaria, leishmaniasis,filariasis and Chagas disease, TB makes part of the high impact neglected diseases, which unfortunately represent an insufficient market to attract enough investment on research by the pharma industry [20]. Whereas the most advanced societies have increased their life expectation thanks to technological development of medicine, in developing countries these diseases (some of which are preventable, treatable, and curable) still devastate the frailest populations. However, governments, multilateral organizations, and foundations spend billions of dollars in the procurement of treatments; and with the current situation of the disease, world health care organisms applaud recent efforts to develop new anti-TB drugs, even though the panorama is not that promising yet [3,21].

5. Platform for the development of active principles in the treatment of TB

Both basic and clinical pharmacology have contributed to the progress in the discovery of drugs applying their experience to the development and validation of hypotheses of new action targets in order to produce novel drugs. In this sense, researchers need to be innovative and they must have a wide vision over the interpretation of the results [20]. The choice of a therapeutic candidate is probably the most important decision to make in the discovery and development of a medication. The chemical structure of a drug confers its biologic, pharmacokinetic, physicochemical, and toxicological properties [22]. On the other hand, the discovery and development of new drugs is a complex and costly process requiring large amount of resources and time. The cost of launching a new drug to the market ranges from US$ 800 million and 1000 million, and it may take between 8 and 17 years depending on the disease and the treatment (Figure 2) [23].

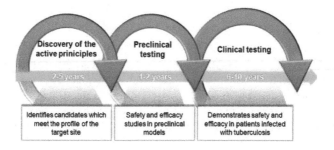

Figure 2. TB drug pipeline. From the discovery bench through preclinical and clinical studies for novel anti-TB agents, a process that could last more than 15 years.

The term "hit" is used to describe a small number of structurally related molecules possessing an established biologic (antituberculosis) activity [24,25]. The term "lead" is defined as a molecule belonging to a series, which shows a substantial structure – activity improvement around a determined *"hit"*, and from which other important factors have been obtained such as evidence of selectivity and pharmacokinetic data or *in vivo* activity [24].

Once these terms are defined it is important to know the biochemical target on which a certain structural type of a chemical compound exerts a biological action. The determination of the mechanism can be carried out *in vitro* by generating drug-resistant mutants which are examined on their whole-genome sequences analysis. The transcriptional profile using cutting edge mycobacterial microarrays or *q*PCR) can be interrogated among the whole transcriptome for potentially distinguishing a defined set of genes involved in the response against chemical injury. Once a determined protein or receptor has been identified, cloning, over-expressing and purifying the proteins is usually performed with the aim of examining its biochemistry and its possibility of affinity or interaction in the tube test is always possible option. Gene deletions and over-expressing systems in *Mycobacterium* are also used for confirming the mechanism of action of a defined candidate [26].Ideally, an antibacterial agent must show bactericidal activity often impeding an essential function for the survival of the microorganism.

Another more classical possibility is monitoring of microbiologic parameters such as growth rate, CFU counting and chemical analysis of metabolites in the treatment with sib MIC, MIC and over-MIC values of the agent. Currently, many active principles are identified as the result of a rational design, supported by genomics inspired hypotheses or from another perspective, by automated high-throughput screening (HTS) using compounds libraries [23].

6. Discovery of active compounds

The parameter most commonly determined to examine the in vitro antibacterial activity of a specific moleculeis the minimum inhibitory concentration (MIC) which represents the concentration required to inhibit 99.9% of the growth of bacilli The main limitations of these trials is that do not describe the percentage of dead bacteria (which critically depends on cell density) or the metabolic state of the bacteria, if we aim to examine the persistent antimicrobial effects of a certain drug [27]. Most publications include at least a compound with a MIC lower than 6.25 mg/Ll [24,26]. It is recommended that active compounds under a colorimetric assay (Resazurin, Alamar Blue, MTT) are reconfirmed usingagar-based techniques or MGIT. A simple and easy to use, agar-based method using Middlebrook 7H10 was introduced in 2004 by Bhakta et al for measuring MIC values [28,29]. The spot culture growth inhibition assay (SPOTi) has now being used to screen more at least more than 1000 compounds. Simultaneously, the cytotoxicity in different type of mammalian and/or macrophages is carried out. The selectivity index (SI) is determined by dividing the growth inhibitory concentration 50 (GIC$_{50}$) corresponding to the concentration of compound capable of killing half of the mammalian cellsby the MIC using the same concentration units. If the SI is larger than 10, infection of a macrophage with a selected strain of mycobacteria and treating with the drug candidate can help to determine its intracellular potential (Figure3)[26].

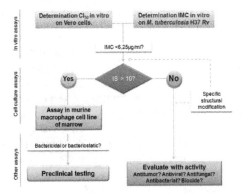

Figure 3. Research and development of new TB active compounds. In an attempt to promote quickly pre-clinical studies of early leads, Orme propose this rapid diagram based on the selectivity ration between a bacteria and mammalian cell line [26].

The macrophage infectionmodel offers the possibility of evaluating the compound in a physiologically challenging intracellular space. By plotting a viability curve fordifferent concentrations of the active principle, The EC_{90}, EC_{99} and $EC_{99.9}$values of are determined verifying the concentration that is able to reduce the bacterial load by 1, 2 and 3 logarithmic units. MIC is most usually defined as EC_{99}.(or EC_{95}). Bactericidal compounds are generally associated with a 3-fold reduction in CFU logarithmic units. In addition the infection assay determines the activity of a compound in an intracellular medium which does not always correlate with *in vitro* media-based inhibition measurements. For instance, transport mechanisms in the cell may influence the intracellular concentration of the drug regardless of the external fluid concentration [30].

The success of a discovery program of antibacterial principles is founded on three factors: identification of key elements contributing to pathogenicity of the microorganism, the understanding of the existing relationships between the microbe and the host, and important-ly, the properties of the chemical compound [30]. Two pathways have been traced with the aim of discovering active principles. One is the empirical pathway, mainly based on chemistry and phenotypic screening; and the more modern is the mechanistic, based on genomics, biochemistry and molecular biology. The former begins with the identification of an active principle with potent antimicrobial activity on *in vitro* conditions. The active principle is discovered by chance or by random screening. Then, it is subject to trial on rigoroustoxico-logical assays before using animal models. Some candidates may eventually beselected for human trials. The limitation of the empirical pathway is the lack of information on the specific target or the action mode, sometimes this lack of understanding can led to high failure rates mostly for toxicity problems [30]. On the other hand,the mechanistic pathway started with the age of molecular biology and genomics which allowed the identification of specific targets of the microbe, absent or structurally different in human hosts. This strategy can be upgradeto high-throughput screening (HTS) platform and to evaluate a large amount a substances in little time. Crystallization of the target proteins and X-ray diffraction spectroscopy, together with an analysis of the active site in the presence of the natural substrate and inhibitors allow the detailed study of the crucial structural interactions.

In the mechanistic approach discovery usually involves firstly the identification and validation of amycobacterial target macromolecule to be inhibited or interrupted. Obtain-ing the small molecules which inhibit such a target is another story. Large collections of compounds can be screened directly against the protein if a high-throughput method of assay is available. Alternatively if there is structural information it is possible to computationally interrogate the target against a defined set of computer-based compounds (docking). The preferred targets are generally the ones ocurring in *M. tuberculosis* and not represented in the human genome. By means of comparative genomics, the targets are present in the human genome. For example, nicotinamide adenine dinucleotide (NAD)is generated in humans either by *de novo*biosynthesis, or by DNA and RNA degradation. However*M. tuberculo-sis*can only synthesize NAD using the*de novo* synthesis. This allows to rationally explorequi-nolinatephosphoribosyltransferase (QAPRTase) inhibition (*de novo* pathway) for the developing of microbial selective inhibitors [30].

Targets existing in *M. tuberculosis*whileabsent in other bacteria would seem ideal since active compounds against this target will be harmless to bacteria beneficial for the human being. However, selecting targets complying with this requisite leads to restrict extensively the likely targets: for the most of it only the biosynthesis of the mycobacterial cell- wall or those implied in specific mycobacterial process (virulence, detoxification, others).

The validation of a target, involves the examination of bacterial viability when decreasingthe protein expression. If reducing the enzyme level,led to lose in bacterial viability, then the target is known as "vulnerable", and it is meant to be attacked [30]. The elimination or knockout of the gene that codifies an essential protein is difficult (or impossible) to produce by homologous recombination if the gene is essential in the conditions of growth, and therefore inducible promoters are a better chance to show the effect of tightly reducing its expression. Over-expression of the target is also possible, the growth of the over-expressed mutant being rescued under higher concentrations of inhibitor. These studied have led to many targets that have been identified and validated. The studies of Sasettiet al identified which enzymes were essential in vitro and in vivo using a transposon site hybridization analysis (TraSH) using both in vitro or in vivo [31,32].

Another approach is related to the genomics of virulence. Some mycobacterial genes are only expressed in granulomabut not inside the macrophages. Isocitratelyase enzyme is fundamental in the persistence of bacilli in chronic infection in mice and its function is related to obtaining carbon during its persistence in the host [8,33]. The extracellular repetition protein (Erp) is another essential protein involved in *M. tuberculosis* virulence that was the first discovered virulence factor. The mutant Δ-erp that does not express correctly the extracellular repetition protein does not show any alteration in standard *in vitro* culture, but maintains an essential function for *in vivo* survival [34,35]. This protein is also a potential target for the development of anti-TB active principles. Two independent proteins (fadD28 and mmpL7) have been identified contributing to the early growth of *M. tuberculosis* in mice lungs and are related to the synthesis and transport of a complex lipid associated to the cell wall, i.e. phthioceroldi-mycocerosate (PDIM) [34]. Although the function of this lipid is unknown, it is suspected that itplays a role in the decrease of the host's immune response. There is no doubt about the remarkable progress that the sequencing of the*M. tuberculosis*genomehas brought to the anti-TB drug discovery area of research. The functional annotation of all these genes remains a considerable amount of experimental work. Sequencing of other related organisms such as *M. marinum, M. leprae, M. aurum*and othersoffer often clues about the essentiality of specific set of genes and operon distribution.

7. Target or compound type in discovery stage

Analogues of thiolactomycin: Thiolactomycinwas the first natural thiolactonedisplaying antibiotic activity. The compound showed moderate *in vitro* activity of 56 μM against *M. tuberculosis*[36]. Thiolactomycin analogues have been synthesized and some hits were found [5]. Analogues of thiolactomycin seem to inhibit mycolatesynthetase, an enzyme involved in the cell wall biosynthesis.

Nitrofuranilamides:*M. tuberculosis*has been found to be susceptible to compounds containing a nitro group. Nitrofuranilamide was identified in a screening for inhibitors of UDP-galacto-semutase [5]. A set of compounds structurally related to nitrofuranilamides was synthesized and tested for antimicrobial activity. All resulted active both to sensitive and resistant strains with a MIC ranging from 0.0004 – 0.05 mg/L [37]. Four nitrofuranilamide type compounds showed significant activity in the tuberculous infection in mice models [37].

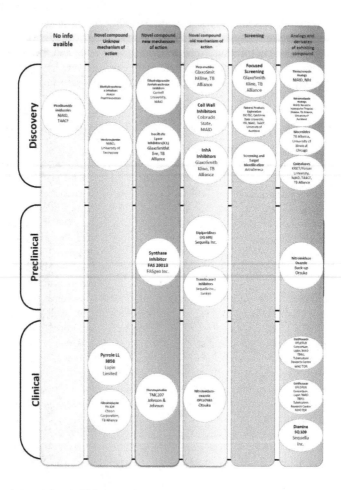

Figure 4. Development of new active compounds targeting *M. tuberculosis*

Analogues of nitroimidazole: While the PA-824 product is developed, the TB Alliance started a project to maximize the potential of this class, by identifying the improved versions of PA-824 [38,39].

Dihydrolipoamideacetyltransferase inhibitors: Dihydrolipoamideacetyltransferase (dlaT) enzyme of *M. tuberculosis* is a potential target for TBdrug discovery [5]. This enzyme is a component of the pyruvate dehydrogenase sub-unit, an enzyme catalyzing acetyl-CoA synthesis and also contributes to peroxinitritereductase, adefense enzyme against oxidative/nitrosative stress. Some heterocyclic compounds have been found to be inhibitors of the dlaT enzyme, displaying non-replicative bacterial killing [40].

"Focused Screening": TB Alliance is helping to develop a set of projects identify chemical compounds which are active against specific molecular targets including DNA gyrase inhibitors (fluoroquinolones targets), peptidedeformylase inhibitors, and quinone-analogous electron transport inhibitors [5].

InhA inhibitors: InhA is the well-known enoyl-reductase of *M. tuberculosis*being an essential-biocatalyst forlong chain fatty acids biosynthesis (FAS-II) [41]. INH resistance is mainly mediated by mutations on KatG, the enzyme activating the prodrug. Consequently, InhA inhibitors that do not require activation by KatGcould be interesting candidates. The main goal of the screening is directInhA inhibition. Some compounds of the biphenylether type have proven to be inhibitory of InhAin a degree correlatingwith*in vitro* growth inhibition [42]. A possible limitation of this class is the possibility of cross resistance with INH and potentially with ETH [5].

Isocitratelyase inhibitors: The isocitratelyase enzyme (ICL) has been found to be essential for the long term persistence of *M. tuberculosis* in mice but not in culture medium or under hypoxia conditions. McKinney and colleagues have proved recently that inhibition of the ICL1 and ICL2 isoforms block bacterial growth and survival in macrophages [8]. The absence of orthologues in mammals for this enzyme, makes it a good target for the development of inhibitors [5]. A screening of more than 900,000 compounds has been performed without satisfactory results. The potential of traditional Chinese medicine has also been researched in obtaining specific inhibitors of this enzyme [43].

Pleuromutilins: Pleuromutilins represent a new kind of antibiotics derived from pleuromu-tiline, a bioactive diterpene initially isolated from edible *Clitopilusscyphoides*fungus [44]. These molecules interfere with protein synthesis associating to the 23S rRNA unit. Despite the structural novelty of these compounds, recent studies have pointed out cross-resistance among pleuromutilins and oxazolidinones[5]. Pleuromutilins have proved to inhibit *M. tuberculosis* growth of *in vitro.*

Macrolides: This project aimed to optimize the anti-TB activity of the macrolide class through the synthesis of modified derivates of erythromycin [5]. Derivatives of erythromycin such as 11, 12-diol, 11, 12-carbamates, and 11, 12-carbazates have been found to be to most promissory [45].

Quinolones and DNA gyrase inhibitors. The goal of this projectwasto synthesize and assess the potential of novel quinolones trying to decrease the time of treatment. More than 450 compounds were synthesized and assessed [5]. The 2-pyridones class has proven to be active DNA gyrase of *M. tuberculosis*, being KR1-10018 an interesting lead for the development of anti-TBdrugs [46].

Survey of natural products: Natural products represent an alternative for the search of new compounds. Different research institutescontinuously carry out screening of natural products (products from plants, fungi, and bacteria) with the hope of identifying compounds with anti-TB activity [5]. Some natural substances have shown significant anti-TB activity: saringosterol 24-epimers, esgosterol-5,8-endoperoxide, micromolide, ascididemin, the manzamines, and engelhardione, among others; however, there is lack of more research regarding selectivity and toxicity [47-50].

Plants: Drugs based on plants extracts have been used worldwide for the treatment of several diseases from ancient times.A great interest in phytomedicine and natural product structures are screened in order to measure their pharmacologic activity. In Colombia, there has been a resurgent interest in the discovery of novel natural anti-TB drugs [50-54].

Natural sea products: oceans are outstanding sources of natural products, not only in invertebrate species such as sponges, mollusks, bryozoos, but also in marine bacteria and marine sediments. The alkaloid (+)-8-hydroxymanzamine A was initially isolated from the *Pachypelli-nasp* sponge[55].In the same way, irciniol A was found in sponges from the Indian Pacific proving to be a good candidate for further studies [56]. Aerothiononine isolated from the marine sponge *Aplysinagerardogreeni*marine sponge was active against clinical isolates of MDR-TB, despite of the resistance patterns, with MIC from 6.5 to 25 mg/L [57]. The alkaloid (+)-8-hydroxymanzamine A alkaloid showed potent inhibitory activity against *M. tuberculosis* H37Rv [58].

Insects. The immune system of invertebrates and vertebrates is made up by cytolitic peptides which act as antimicrobial agents during the invasion of eukaryotes and prokaryotes microorganisms. Poison from arachnids (spiders and scorpions) contains toxic peptides of high molecular weight (2 – 12 kDa) with high specificity against prokaryote cells [59]. This type of compounds may be very promising as a drug in the treatment of tuberculosis.

Microorganisms. Most of the major antibiotics drugs have been isolated frommicroorganisms. Streptomycin,the first effective anti-TB drug was identified in *Streptomyces griseus*. Besides streptomycin, aminogyicosides kanamycin, amikacin, and capreomycinhave been very important therapeutically as second-line agents [59]. Other important anti-TB drugs in TB treatment are the rifamycins, which constitute a group of semi-synthetic antibiotics isolated from *Streptomyces mediterrani*[59].

8. Preclinical and clinical development for new anti-tuberculosis drugs

8.1. Preclinical development of anti-TB active principles

Preclinical tests involve the use of animal models to prove the efficacy and safety of a given candidate before being tested in humans. Because of its management in terms of size, offer, maintenance, strength, and reproducibility, the mouse constitutes the preferred animal model for *in vivo* research of the TB infection [60]. Other possible animal models include rats, guinea pigs, and macaques. The amounts of viable mycobacteria and mortality and the possibility of organomegaly in the pulmonary tissue are evaluated during therapy, at the end of therapy and in the post-therapy period. Post antibiotic effect, relapses, and resistance development are examined. Antagonists, additives, or synergistic effects are also evaluated when the compound is administered in combination with other active principles, as well as its capability to sterilize lesions in experimentally infected animals. Finally, toxicological studies, which must be highly controlled and documented, are carried out forthe determination of the safety window in order to perform the subsequent clinical trials in humans [60].

The drugs regime must be administered for several months, using commonly between 100 – 150 mice per test, therefore requiring large amounts of space and resources for maintaining the animals. Model in mice is more effective regarding the cost-benefit relation, and most of the data obtained can be reproduced in clinical studies. The model of infection by TB in mice has served to predict the sterilizing potential of new compounds, the effectiveness of the combination of drugs, success in intermittent therapy and the duration of therapy necessary to avoid relapse. The effectiveness of the active principle is measured mainly the reduction of the colony forming units (CFU) in the lung and spleen. Several varieties of mice have been used in laboratories conducting this type of test and, to this date, no comparisons have been reported [61].

Genetically modified mice have been used in the in bioassay of compounds with anti-mycobacterial activity [62]. A mouse that does not express the interferon-γ gene (knock-out) is incapable of producing cytokine Th1 and therefore suffers a more acute infection. Bioassay with this mouse allows determining the initial efficacy of a chemical compound in six days. Because of their statistical power, substances with low antimycobacterial activity can be detected by a small decrease in the CFU count. The model has great usefulness in initial trials, when there is a limited amount of the chemical compound. Another model, still under development, has been proposed to study relapse. An animal that cannot produce the granulocyte-macrophage-colony stimulation factor (GM-CSF) is used.

Wayne's model, which indicates the effect of compounds against persistent bacilli, has also been used. Bacilli under anoxia conditions are used and they are directly inoculated in the mouse. The guinea pig model also allows observing the destruction of tissue by caseous necrosis where there is not oxygen contribution and bacteria go into a hypoxia state [61].

Pharmacokinetics and pharmacodynamics range from *in vitro* tests, *in vivo* tests in animal models, and finally clinical trials in humans [57]. The simplest pharmacodynamic measure is determining the MIC *in vitro*, used widely in the primary discovery of active principles. This measure can be roughly related to the maximum cut point of the active principle concentration in plasma (C_{max}) and can aid in the prediction of *in vivo* pharmacodynamics among a series of structurally related agents. However, it does not represent the concentration at which the growth ceases, and, as we have already seen, does not allow distinguishing between bacteri-cide and bacteriostatic activity. Moreover, it does not allow obtaining information regarding the dynamic relationships *in vivo* either, since the growth conditions do not represent the ones of persistent organisms in the living tissue.

Animal models enable to evaluate the *in vivo* efficacy of novel active principles regimens. Protection experiments using monotherapyfor a certain amount of time and then performing lethal intravenous or aerosol inoculation can prove the efficacy and selection of a preliminary dose. Studies on the short term using colonies count in different homogenized organs allow estimating the bactericide capability of a medication or a combination of drugs, as well as the likely appearance of resistance [57]. However, in order to describe the sterilizing activity of a given compound, a larger study time is required as well as other techniques since negative cultures finalizing the therapy do not necessarily indicate that there was sterilization. Three months are required after the end of treatment to determine a durable cure and success of the sterilization. Cornell's mouse model uses an intensive therapy in order to obtain negative cultures and then evaluate the ability of individual active principles or their combinations to prevent relapse when the mouse is left untreated or when it is maintained immunocompromised[57].

The following are the PK and PD parameters which are calculated in the trial with mice: the C/MIC quotient, defined as the ratio of the serum maximum concentration (C_{max}) over the MIC; the AUC/MIC quotient, defined as the ratio of the area below the concentration-time curve (AUC) over the MIC in the serum during the total time of treatment(144 h) divided by 6 in order to obtain a daily value (AUC_{24}/MIC); and the percentage of time above the MIC (T > MIC) estimated by the first order kinetic equation $C = C_0\, e^{-kt}$, where C_0 is the concentration to time 0, k is the constant and t the time, and it is defined as the percentage of the 144-hour time in which the medication concentration surpasses the MIC in the serum [63].

Recent studies of the PK and PD parameters for INH, RIF, and fluoroquinolones have improved the understanding of PK and PD properties of these drugs. Although the PK and PD parameters are characterized for antibacterial agents, a clear description of the efficacy is still lacking [63]. The parameter that best describes the bactericidal activity of anti-TB drugs in the mice model is AUC_{24} / MIC, with a correlation of 0.83. For INH when the value of AUC_{24} / MIC reaches 500, the maximum effect is observed with a decrease of 1.3 log CFU per mouse lung. In other words, the INH effect was the same when the total doses were administered into 6, 12, or 18 doses divided equally during one week [63]. Mitchison observed that the administration of a single total dose of INH in infected guinea pigs had the same effect than if administered daily, every other day, or every four days during a six-week period. Therefore, the efficacy of INHwas dependent on the size of the doses but not on the regime [63]. Preclinical trials that establish pharmacodynamic and pharmacokinetic properties enable to obtain information regarding the optimal doses and regimens.

Despite of the large use of the mouse model,this rodentdoes not develop the typical human lesions observed in pulmonary TB such as caseous necrosis or cavitations[57]. Also, one has to be very prudent conducting escalation in the doses of the agents between the mouse and the human due to the metabolic differences and possible pharmacokinetic interactions. The histological characteristics of guinea pigs in a TB infection are more similar to human pathology; but there is little experience in the chemotherapeutical use of this model. Preliminary studies suggest that the guinea pig model is capable of differentiating the sterilizing activities of INH and RIF [57].

A good model to study latent forms of TB is the cynomolgus macaque (*Macacafascicularis*) [61, 64]. All primates infected by bronchial instillation developed the infection, based on the tuberculin test and immune responses to *M. tuberculosis* antigens. Differences in the progression of the disease for the 17 macaques studied were observed. Between 50 – 60% of infected primates developed active and chronic infection, characterized by clear signs of disease in thoracic x-rays and other tests. Approximately 40% of the initially infected macaques did not develop the disease in the 20 months of study. These primates showed clinical signs of latent TB. In summary, the study proves that it is possible to use the cynomolgus macaque in infection by *M. tuberculosis* because it presents the complete spectrum of infection in humans (rapid and lethal infection, chronic infection, and latent infection). This animal model is the only one that enables to study the latent forms of the infection. Its great advantage is the high pathologic similarity of the infection in macaques and humans, whereas the disadvantages are the cost and maintenance of the animals, particularly since they require facilities with Biosafety Level 3 [64]. This model has been proposed in final preclinical trials for the development of active principles for latent forms of TB [61].The following are examples of promising compounds in preclinical phase. Some of these substances are protected by patents and therefore access to information is restricted.

The following are examples of promising compounds in preclinical phase. Some of these substances are protected by patents and therefore access to information is restricted.

SQ609 dipiperidine: this compound is a completely novel anti-TB active principle. It acts by interrupting the biosynthesis ofcell wall, but its specific mechanism is unknown [5]. It demonstratedantymycobacterial activity in an*in vivo* mouse model.

FAS20013 synthetase ATP inhibitor: Inhibition of bacterial fatty acids synthesis (FASII) still represents a valid, target for the discovery of anti-TBdrugs. However, this novel compound was identified by Fasgen and it has as action target the inhibition of enzymes for biosynthesis of fatty acids in *Mycobacterium* [65]. It belongs to the β-sulfonylcarboxamides class.

Translocase inhibitors SQ641: The pharmaindustryis developing a series of translocase inhibitors for the treatment of TB. The mycobacterial translocase I is an enzyme required for the biosynthesis of the cell wall, and the SQ641 compound has been reported as a selective inhibitor of this enzyme [66,67].

8.2. Clinical development of anti-TB active principles

Identifying new anti-TB is a complex and highly regulated process carried out around a critical moment: when the new compound is tested in humans [5]. Currently, clinical images offer a support method for generation of drugs which enables to establish information about the bio-distribution of the molecule, interaction of the target, and pharmacokinetics[68]. Clinical development of a promising substance is usually divided into four phases. The first phase is carried out in healthy human beings and it provides information regarding the chemical compound pharmacokinetic profile, and some preliminary information regarding safety [69]. Phase I trials are conducted in a small size, usually 15 to 30 subjects, and can be of single or multiple doses. Besides the phase I trials, researchers may consider incorporating the phar-macokinetics and safety studies to a wider population size (200 to 300 subjects). Phase II studies are conducted on patients diagnosed with active TB. The efficacy in monotherapy and combination therapy is evaluated. One of the objectives of trials in phase I/II is to determine the optimal dose for the phase III studies.

Early Bactericidal Activity (EBA) is one of the fundamental parameters to determine the clinical efficacy of active principles [70]. It consists on a large trial conducted on patients recently diagnosed with pulmonary TB who are treated with active principles or combinations for a period of 2 to 14 days. Patients must not have used anti-TB drugs previously. During the treatment period, the amount of viable bacilli appearing in sputum samples is determined quantitatively. The traditional EBA unit is the logarithmic decrease of colony forming units (CFU/mL sputum/day during the first 48 hours). EBA studies have shown that there are differences between the fall of viable bacteria counts in the first two days of treatment in comparison with the following twelve [71]. Differences among several treatments were also more significant during the first two days. In the early therapy, the activity of INH was superior and dominant regarding the other active principles administered in combination. Any addition of INH to a regime leads to an increase of EBA but never higher than INH on its own. The addition of PZA to a regime of STR, INH, and RIF increased 0-2 days EBA from 0.415 to 0.472 [71]. The greatest disadvantage of determining the EBA is its inability to detect sterilizing activity. Some researchers have concluded that extended EBA trials (2 to 14 days) do not correlate to the sterilizing activity [72]. For example, the potent sterilizing activity of PZA was not detected in an extended EBA trial. STR showed potent activity in extended EBA, and it is known it has a very low sterilizing activity in randomized clinical trials. In extended EBA, EMB appears as antagonist; however, there is no clinical evidence that this drug interferes with the sterilizing effects of RIF and PZA [72].

In order to determine the sterilizing activity of the anti-TB active principles, and 8-week study has been proposed, and the ratio of patients whose sputum be negative is determined; this parameter correlates to the ratio of patients who suffer relapse after the treatment [73]. In these studies, frequent counts of the number of viable bacilli are carried out being known as "serial sputum CFU counts" or SSCC. This method enables to distinguish between differences in the organisms that divide rapidly from the persistent ones. These studies turn out to be appropriate to determine the possibility of a regime to decrease the time of treatment [73].

Phase III clinical trials are carried out at large scale; they are randomized and they are conducted to demonstrate the improved or equivalent efficacy of a new treatment against standard treatments [60]. Around 1000 patients are enrolled per study for TB and the cure on treated patients is bacteriologically observed during certain amount of time as well as the ratio of relapse. The accepted end point to demonstrate efficacy is 2 years. The experimental design of Phase III trials must be designed cautiously clearly definingcritical primary and secondary end points, the size of the sample, the intervalsof confidence, and the statistical methods that will be used to obtain the data [60]. It is fundamental that microbiologic assessments are being conducted during an appropriate time, with the aim of determining the real activity of the researched agent. To ensure a sufficient population in Phase III studies, trials may be conducted in countries with high incidence rate of TB. Countries possessing a robust and expansive TB control program that provides essential information such as annual incidence (location of the disease, comorbility, resistance) are preferred. A reference laboratory is required for most of

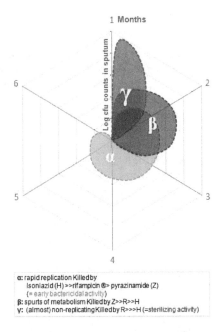

α: rapid replication Killed by
Isoniazid (H) >>rifampicin ®> pyrazinamide (Z)
(= early bactericidal activity)
β: spurts of metabolism Killed by Z>>R>>H
γ: (almost) non-replicating Killed by R>>>H (=sterilizing activity)

Figure 5. Pharmacological activity of RIF, INH and PZA targeting *M. tuberculosis* subpopulations. Differential population of *M. tuberculosis* in the lesions, observed after 6 months of treatment.as log CFU in sputum

the trials, but there is also need to extend duplicates to local laboratories. Finally, validated relapse markers, which provide evidence of the sterilizing activity of an active principle or regime, are used. To this end, the most used method is determining the ratio of patients who have a negative sputum culture, 8 weeks after the beginning of the treatment compared to the standard treatment. Molecular methods using relapse markers require greater study and validation in order to be employed successfully [60].

Phase IV studies include product development efforts such as patents, description of biologic activity, toxicity, safety profile in humans and demonstrated clinical efficacy. Best manufacturing practices studies are conducted, as well as laboratory and clinical practice to ensure the marketing needs of the product. Post-marketing studies duringPhase IV are typically assessment of new regimens in comparison to thenormally used, and surveillance of likely adverse effects, including the development of resistance. The acceptance for use of the new active principle must be subscribed by the patient, and the economic benefits of the new drug must also be established [60].

SQ109 diamine: The lead was identified in a screening conducted in 2003 using a combinatory library based on EMB as pharmacophore. It shows an MIC value of 0.11 μg/ml. t remains equally active as EMB at 100 mg/kg when administered in the mouse model at a dose of 1 mg/kg. However, SQ109 did not increase its effectiveness at higher doses (10 mg/kg, 25 mg/kg) and it was clearly less effective than INH[5]. Its effectiveness has been proved against MDR strains. Preclinical toxicology studies have been completed and further phase II clinical studies are underway [67].

TMC-207 diarylquinoline: This agent is a promising agent as a new kind of antimycobacterial agent. Twenty diarylquinolines have been reported on the series with MIC lower than 0.5 mg/L against H_{37}Rv. Antimycobacterial activity was confirmed *in vivo* for three compounds of this class. The most effective agent was TMC-207, which had a MIC of 0.06 mg/L against H_{37}Rv and its spectrum was unique in specificity against mycobacteria [74]. TMC-207 inhibits the ATP synthetase leading to a decrease of ATP and a pH imbalance. This compound has a potent EBA in the murine infection model, superior or similar to INH. The combinations TMC-207, INH, and PZA cleansed the bacilli present in the lungs of all mice after two months. Trials have also been conducted in mice with combinations of second line agents. Preliminary studies have proved *in vivo* sterilizing activity in the mice model, and decrease in the treatment time. Currently it is in phase IIa. Therefore, it is the most promising drug candidate in the last 30 years.

Gatifloxacin: It has been reported bactericidal activity *in vitro* and *in vivo* against *M. tuberculosis* to this compound. Its MIC has been reported between 0.25 mg/L and 0.03 mg/L against H_{37}Rv [76]. In an *in vitro* study on bacilli in stationary phase, gatifloxacin showed the greatest bactericidal activity in the first two days, but none afterwards. In mice studies, the combination of gatifloxacin with EMB and PZA cleansed the lungs of infected animals after two months of treatment. Currently, gatifloxacin is under phase III to prove the efficacy and safety of a four-month regime for the treatment of pulmonary TB supervised by the European Commission Oflotub Consortium, WHO-TDR, Tuberculosis Research Unit (TBRU), National Institute of Allergy and Infectious Diseases (NIAID), Tuberculosis Research Centre [5,67].

Moxifloxacin: Moxifloxacin is the most promising fluorquinolone against *M. tuberculosis*. Its activity *in vitro* seems to affect bacilli unaffected by RIF. Its MIC reported *in vitro* is 0.5 mg/L [77]. It seems that moxifloxacin interferes with the protein synthesis on bacteria with low metabolic activity by a mechanism different to the one of RIF. However, the specific action mechanism is unknown. In the mouse model, the effectiveness of moxifloxacin is comparable to INH. When administered in combination with PZA, moxifloxacin has a greater bactericidal activity tan the INH + RIF + PZA regime. In fact, the combination RIF + moxifloxacin + PZA decreases completely bacilli count within four months, whereas the combination RIF + INH + PZA requires 6 months. It is likely that there is synergism among the three drugs, and the alternative regime replacing INH by moxifloxacin has been proposed. Moxifloxacin is under phase III [67]. Clinical studies have not proved a greater sterilizing activity of a regime containing moxifloxacin in comparison with the standard regime; however, it has increased activity in early points [5,75].

Nitroimidazole PA-824: This bicyclical nitroimidazole is under development by the TB Alliance, which has the proprietary rights. The *in vitro* MIC of the PA-824 compound is between 0.15 and 0.3 µg/ml [78].After an activation by the F420 factor of *M. tuberculosis*, the PA-824 compound inhibits biosynthesis of the cell wall components by means of mechanisms still to be established. It has proved bactericidal activity against replicative and static bacilli *in vitro*. Although PA-824 was more efficient than INH or moxifloxacin, during the continuation phase it was not better than the RIF + INHH combination. On the long term, the 12-month treatment did not achieve total eradication in any of the mice treated. The 6-month regime of PA-824 in combination with RIF, INH, and PZA in mice proved to be superior to the standard regime regarding quickness of eradication and lower relapse rate. This compound has been widely evaluated in animals and humans; currently it is under phase II clinical trials as part of an initial scheme (PA-824, moxifloxacin, and PZA) containing new anti-TB drugs[79].

Nitroimidazole-oxazol OPC67683: There is very little public information regarding this compound. It belongs to a subclass of mycolic acids synthesis inhibitors. It has shown *in vitro* activity against standard and resistant strains, showing a MICof 12 ng/ml [80]. It has not shown cross resistance with any other medication. The compound shown activity against bacilli residing within human macrophages and type II pneumocytes. The chronic TB trial in mice demonstrated an activity 6 – 7 times more effective than the one observed for first line INH and RIFdrugs. Favorable oral absorption and distribution have been reported. Currently it is under phase II clinical trials.

Pyrrole LL-3858: Some pyrroles derivatives have been found to have *in vitro* activity against *M. tuberculosis*. The MIC of pyrrole LL-3858 is between 0.025 and 0.12 µg/ml. The LL-3858 derivate identified by Lupin Limited showed greater bactericidal activity in the lungs of mice infected in monotherapy than INH. The trial of LL-3858 in combination with INH and RIF, or with INH, RIF, and PZA sterilized the totality of mice in 3 months [5]. Currently, the compound is under phase II clinical trials [67].

8.3. New approaches for the development of anti-TB active principles

In the dawn of the 21st century, pathogenesis of the infectious disease appears as a competition between the host and the pathogen involving short term adaptations and co evolution of the genomes [81]. The pathogen and the host constantly exercise selective pressure over each other, making the environment in test tube completely different from that within the host.

In latent tuberculous infection (LTBI), most of bacilli are not replicating, whereas in a phase of active disease most of the population is on active growth. Chemotherapy must take this metabolic adversity to favor the host.A durable cure must eliminate both the replicative and the persistent bacilli.Eradication of the persistent bacilli onchemotherapylasting between 6 – 24 months has been proposed in order to avoid relapse. However, such a long treatment is difficult to sustain and there is always resistance-associated risks in interrupted regimens [81].A philosophy of mycobacterial infection states that the essential genes for infection in mice include genes that are not essential *in vitro*.

The proteasome of *M. tuberculosis* is a set of proteins that provide a quick adaptation to changing conditions [82]. Two genes, *mpa* (*Mycobacterium* proteosomal ATPase) and *pafA* (proteasome accessory factor) were identified as important in the survival of *M. tuberculosis*to exposure against reactive nitrogen species (RNS) *in vitro* and required for active disease *in vivo* [82]. These genes codify for proteins involved in the bacteria proteasomal function. Proteasomes are barrel-shaped proteases consisting of 14 α units and 14 β units [82]. Mpa is similar to ATPases found in the proteosome of eukaryotes cells, and chemical inhibition of the protease activity of the *M. tuberculosis* proteosome causes sensitization of the wild strain to reactive nitrogen species (RNS). The PafA protein does not share homology with any protein of known function [82]. Two specific proteasomeinhibitors, epoxomicin and a peptidic-boronate prevented the growth of *M. tuberculosis* and turned out to be bactericidal during the recovery of the mycobacterium against exposure to RNS [81]. The operon that codifies for the proteasome was knocked out by using conditional gene silencing and it was proved that bacteria require it to survive during the chronic infection in mice and its silencing allowed the mouse to be free of the persistent infection [83]. Whereas the proteasome of the mycobacterium is essential for the infection of a host, it is not required to grow in a rich and aerated medium such as Middlebrook 7H9 broth [81].

Unlike other bacteria, *M. tuberculosis* possesses a unique defense system that relates the antioxidant and metabolic activities [81]. The system includes a peroxyredoxin, the C subunit of an alkylhydroperoxy-reductase (AhpC), a thioredoxin type protein (AhpD), dihydrolipoa-mideacyltransferase (DlaT), and lipoamide dehydrogenase (Lpd), and the four enzymes together work as peroxydases and peroxynitroreductases and peroxynitroreductasesdepend-ant of NADH [81]. The dual functionality of these enzymes is interesting as potential targets for the development of anti-TB active principles.

Moreover, the DosRsystem,discovered 15 years ago, regulates the development of a form of non-eplicative survival without morphologic differentiation in *M. tuberculosis* (known as latency state). This state of physiologic quiescence maintained viable the microorganism for long periods of time, contributing with two key characteristicsof TB: the symptom-free latent infection state and the persistence of the active disease of the tubercular infection in spite of the prolonged therapy time. Due to the importance of the bacilli latency state in the pathophysiology and chemotherapy of the disease, researchers have set their interest in the DosR system. Drugs that attack the latent state of the bacterium not only would be the key for eradication of the latent infection, but also shortening the time of treatment of active infection [84].

9. A new approach to research processes

Traditionally, the focus of research is the evaluation of a single drugin extensive and costly trials. This process may take a lot of time and reduces the possibility of developing a combi-nation of new drugs that is effective. For this reason, a new approach to research has been led by the Critical Path to TB Drug Regimens (CPTR) organization created in March 2010 by the Bill & Melinda Gates Foundations, the Critical Path Institute, and the TB Alliance. This strategic partnership has the strength of reducing the time necessary to develop a new TB treatment scheme, as well as reducing significantly the research costs. This initiative has been endorsed by the US Food and Drug Administration and other regulatory entities, as well as the World Health Organization [67].

As a result of the 41st Union World Conference in Berlin, Germany, on November 2010, the TB Alliance announced the launch of the first clinical phase to test a new TB treatment scheme which expedites the treatment of patients. The combination of three drugs has been promising for the treatment of drug sensitive (DS-TB) and MDR-TB, thus changing the course of the TB pandemics through simplification and shortening in the treatment time of the disease world-wide. The combination is currently in phase II of clinical trials and contains PA-824 and moxifloxacin together with PZA. Researchers have reported that preclinical data reveal a decrease in the treatment time both for DS-TB and MDR-TB patients, and possibly XDR-TB ones with a simple three-drug treatment scheme [67].

10. Nano-particles: A projection towards the future

Nanoparticles can create new directions in the diagnosis, treatment, and prevention of TB. A significant application in the progress of this technology is using drug carriers.This system has been found to be advantageous, as it gives high stability of the drug, high load capacity (many molecules of the medication can be incorporated in the matrix of the particle), easiness to incorporate hydrophilic and hydrophobic substances, possibility of being administered orally or via inhalation. Perhaps more importantly, the anti-TB drug release in a controlled manner from the matrix enables to improve the bioavailability and reduction of the doses frequency. Load or delivery systems such as liposome or microspheres have been developed for the sustained release of anti-TB drugs, and better chemotherapeutical efficacy has been found when the system is researched in animal models (e.g. mice) [85,86].In 2005, the efficacy of nanoparticles was assessed in the distribution of anti-TBdrugs administered every 10 days versus the non capsulated form of aerosol administration of drugs against *M. tuberculosis* in guinea pigs; in both cases the treatments reduced the bacteria count. These findings suggest that the distribution of drugs by nanoparticles has a great potential in the treatment of TB [86].

11. Conclusions

Currently, devastating diseases in the world such as tuberculosis get the attention of author-ities with the aim of supporting breakthroughs which provide alternatives for their control.

The development of active principles against *M. tuberculosis* is nowadays a worldwide priority due to the appearance of strains resistant to medications used in current therapeutic schemes, thus existing the need to articulate in an expedite manner the basic research looking for new therapeutic choices, along with clinical research and its articulation with the industry in order to guarantee a quick production of novel alternatives which overcome the limitations of current treatment schemes.

The concern in many sectors devoted to tuberculosis control is that there are not sufficient alternatives that can join rapidly the treatment against tuberculosis, and they convey discour-aging estimations regarding the degree of resistance that each one of these molecules will have at the moment of entering the therapeutic scheme deduced from natural resistant bacilli. These justifications have promoted research around the world towards finding new molecules, based on investigations of natural sources such as plants, insects, marine microorganisms, synthetic molecules deduced from the modification or substitutions made on the structure of already existing molecules with the aim of potentiate their effect; or from new sources such as nanoparticles, computing studies, among many others.

The results expected at the end of each process producing a new alternative of treatment against tuberculosis is that these drugs may shorten the duration of the current treatment, be active against resistant strains and non-replicative conditions of *M. tuberculosis* as well as not interfering with HIV antiretroviral therapy, reduce adverse side effects, and that it is of easy administration to facilitate the patient's compliance. For the management of tuberculosis as a public health event worldwide, these new drugs must be produced easily in large amounts; they must be stable under minimum storage conditions, and they must be of low cost so that all governments may guarantee access of all the diseased population.

For these expectations to become true in the short term, more basic and applied research is required to generate new ideas in the development of anti-tuberculosis drugs, as well as stronger financial support in research and greater commitment from the pharmaceutical industry and public health entities.

Acknowledgements

Magda Lorena Orduz and Hernando YesidEstupiñan for the figures and technical contribution to manuscript.

Author details

Juan D. Guzman[1], Ximena Montes-Rincón[2] and Wellman Ribón[2]

1 Subdirección de Investigación, Instituto Nacional de Salud, Bogotá, Colombia

2 Grupo de Inmunología y Epidemiologia Molecular, Universidad Industrial de Santander. Bucaramanga, Colombia

References

[1] World Health Organization. Global Tuberculosis control(2011). WHO Report. 2011.http://www.who.int/tb/publications/global_report/en/index.htmlaccessed   16 september 2012).

[2] Mitnick, C. D, Shin, S. S, Seung, K. J, Rich, M. L, Atwood, S. S, Furin, J. J, et al. Comprehensivetreatment of extensively drug-resistant tuberculosis. N Engl J Med (2008). , 359, 563-74.

[3] Casenghi, M, Cole, S. T, & Nathan, C. F. New approaches to filling the gap in tuberculosisdrug discovery. PLoS Med (2007). e293.

[4] Sacks, L, & Behrman, R. Developing new drugs for the treatment of drug-resistant tuberculosis: a regulatory perspective. Tuberculosis (Edinb). (2008). Suppl 1:S, 93-100.

[5] Casenghi, M. Development of new drugs for TB chemotherapy. In campaign for access to essential medicines. Médecins sans frontiers ((2006). http://www.msf.or.jp/info/pressreport/pdf/TBpipeline_E.pdfaccessed 16 september 2012).

[6] Cantón, R, & Ruiz-garbajosa, P. Co-resistance: an opportunity for the bacteria and resistance genes. Current Opinion in Pharmacology (2011). , 11(5), 477-485.

[7] Ribon, W. Biochemical Isolation and Identification of Mycobacteria. In: Jimenez J. (ed)Biochemical testing. InTech; (2012). Available from http://www.intechop-en.com/books/biochemical-testing/biochemical-isolation-and-identification-of-myco-bacteria, 21-52.

[8] Mckinney, J. D. HonerZuBentrup K, Munoz-Elias EJ, Miczak A, Chen B, Chan WT, et al. Persistence of Mycobacterium tuberculosis in macrophages and mice requires the glyoxylate shunt enzyme isocitratelyase. Nature (2000). , 406-735.

[9] Mitchison, D. A. Basic mechanisms of chemotherapy. Chest. (1979). Suppl) , 771-81.

[10] Jassal, M, & Bishai, W. R. Extensively drug-resistant tuberculosis. Lancet Infect Dis (2009). , 9(1), 19-30.

[11] Raviglione, M. C. Facing extensively drug-resistant tuberculosis- a hope and a challenge. New Engl J Med (2008). , 359, 636-38.

[12] Kidder, T. Mountains Beyond Mountains. Random House Publishing Group. (2009).

[13] Rivers, E. C, & Mancera, R. L. New anti-tuberculosis drugs in clinical trials with novel mechanisms of action. Drug Discov Today (2008).

[14] Castiblanco, C. A, & Ribón, W. Coinfección de tuberculosis en pacientes con VIH/SIDA: un análisis según las fuentes de información en Colombia. Infect (2006). , 10(4), 232-42.

[15] Harries, A. D, Chimzizi, R, & Zachariah, R. Safety, effectiveness, and outcomes of concomitant use of higly active antiretroviral therapy with drugs for tuberculosis in re-source-poor settings. Lancet. (2006). , 367(9514), 944-5.

[16] Corbett, E. L, Martson, B, Churchyard, G. J, & De Cock, K. M. Tuberculosis in sub-SaharanAfrica: opportunities, challenges, and change in the era of antiretroviral treatment.Lancet (2006). , 367(9514), 926-37.

[17] Theuretzbacher, U. Resistance drives antibacterial drug development. CurrOpin-Pharmacol (2011). , 11(5), 433-438.

[18] Nguyen, T. Tuberculosis: a global health emergency, Outlook(1999). , 17, 1-8.

[19] Brien, O. RJ. Development of fluoroquinolones as first-line drugs for Tuberculosis-atlong last, Am. J. Resp. Crit. Care. Med. (2003). , 68, 1266-67.

[20] Trist, D, & Davies, C. How technology can aid the pharmacologist in carrying out drugdiscovery. CurrOpinPharmacol (2011). , 11(5), 494-495.

[21] Pecoul, B. New drugs for neglected diseases: from pipeline to patients, PLoS Med(2004). , 1(1), 19-23.

[22] Rossi, T, & Braggio, S. Quality by Design in lead optimization: a new strategy to ad-dress productivity in drug discovery. CurrOpinPharmacol. (2011). , 11(5), 515-20.

[23] Showalter, H. D, & Denny, W. A. A roadmap for drug discovery and its translation to small molecule agents in clinical development for tuberculosis treatment. Tuberculo-sis (Edinb). (2008). Suppl 1 S, 3-17.

[24] Ballell, L, Field, R. A, Duncan, K, & Young, R. J. New small-molecule synthetic anti-myco- bacterials. AntimicrobAgentsChemother (2005). , 49(6), 2153-63.

[25] Williams, M. (2011). Qualitative pharmacology in a quantitative world: diminishing value in the drug discovery process. CurrOpinPharmacol. 2011;, 11(5), 496-500.

[26] Orme, I. M. Search for new drugs for treatment of tuberculosis. Antimicrob Agents Chemother (2001). , 45, 1943-46.

[27] Singh, R, & Tam, V. Optimizing dosage to prevent emergence of resistance- lessons from in vitro models. CurrOpinPharmacol. (2011). , 11(5), 453-56.

[28] Bhakta, S, et al. ArylamineN-Acetyltransferase Is Required for Synthesis of Mycolic Acids and Complex Lipids in Mycobacterium bovis BCG and Represents a Novel Drug Target. J Exp Med. (2004). , 199(9), 1191-9.

[29] Evangelopoulos, D, & Bhakta, S. Rapidmethods for testinginhibitors of mycobacter-ialgrowth. MethodsMol Biol. (2010). , 642, 193-201.

[30] Balganesh, T. S, Balasubramanian, V, & Kumar, S. A. Drug discovery for tuberculo-sis: bot- tlenecks and path forward. CurrSci (2004). , 86(1), 167-76.

[31] Sassetti, C. M, & Rubin, E. J. Geneticrequirements for mycobacterialsurvival during infection. ProcNatlAcadSci U S A. (2003). , 100(22), 12989-94.

[32] Sassetti, C. M, Boyd, D. H, & Rubin, E. J. Genes required for mycobacterial growth defined by high density mutagenesis. MolMicrobiol. (2003). , 48(1), 77-84.

[33] Murphy, D. J, & Brown, J. R. Novel drug target strategies against Mycobacterium tu-berculosis. CurrOpinMicrobiol (2008). , 11(5), 422-27.

[34] Chopra, P, Meena, L. S, & Singh, Y. New drugs for Mycobacterium tuberculosis. In-dian J Med Res ((2003). , 117, 1-9.

[35] Berthet, F. X, Lagranderie, M, Gounon, P, Laurent-winter, C, Ensergueix, D, Chavarot, P, et al. Attenuation of virulence by disruption of the Mycobacterium tuberculosis erp gene. Science (1998). , 282(5389), 759-762.

[36] Douglas, J. D, Senior, S. J, Morehouse, C, Phetsukiri, B, Campbell, I. B, Besra, G. S, et al. Analogues of thiolactomycin; potential drugs with enhanced anti-mycobacterial activity. Microbiology (2002). , 148(10), 3101-09.

[37] Hurdle, J. G, Lee, R. B, Budha, N. R, Carson, E. I, Qi, J, Scherman, M. S, et al. A microbiologicalassessment of novel nitrofuranylamides as anti-tuberculosis agents. J AntimicrobChemother (2008). , 62(5), 1037-45.

[38] Kim, P, Kang, S, Boshoff, H. I, Jiricek, J, Collins, M, Singh, R, et al. a Structure-activity relationships of antitubercularnitroimidazoles. 2. Determinants of aerobic activity andquantitative structure-activity relationships. J Med Chem (2009). , 52(5), 1329-44.

[39] Kim, P, Zhang, L, Manjunatha, U. H, Singh, R, Patel, S, Jiricek, J, et al. b Structure-activityrelationships of antitubercularnitroimidazoles. 1. Structural features associated withaerobic and anaerobic activities of 4- and 5-nitroimidazoles. J Med Chem (2009). , 52(5), 1317-28.

[40] Bryk, R, Gold, B, Venugopal, A, Singh, J, Samy, R, Pupek, K, et al. Selective killing ofnonreplicating mycobacteria. Cell Host Microbe (2008). , 3(3), 137-45.

[41] Raman, K, Rajagopalan, P, & Chandra, N. Flux balance analysis of mycolic acid pathway:targets for anti-tubercular drugs. PLoSComput Biol. (2005). Oct;1(5)

[42] Lu, H, & Tonge, P. J. Inhibitors of FabI, an enzyme drug target in the bacterial fatty acidbiosynthesis pathway. AccChem Res (2008). , 41(1), 11-20.

[43] Bai, B, Xie, J. P, Yan, J. F, Wang, H. H, & Hu, C. H. A high throughput screening approach toidentify isocitratelyase inhibitors from traditional chinese medicine sources. DrugDevelop Res (2007). , 67(10), 818-23.

[44] Tsukagagoshi, T, Tokiwano, T, & Oikawa, H. Studies on the later stage of the biosynthesis of pleuromutilin. BiosciBiotechnolBiochem (2007). , 71(12), 3116-21.

[45] Falzari, K, Zhu, Z, Pan, D, Liu, H, Hongmanee, P, & Franzblau, S. G. In vitro and in vivoactivities of macrolide derivatives against Mycobacterium tuberculosis. AntimicrobAgents Chemother (2005). , 49(4), 1447-54.

[46] Lenaerts, A. J, Bitting, C, Woolhiser, L, Gruppo, V, Marietta, K. S, Johnson, C. M, & Orme, I. M. Evaluation of a 2-pyridone, KRQ-10018, against Mycobacterium tuberculosis in vitroand in vivo. Antimicrob Agents Chemother (2008). , 52(4), 1513-15.

[47] Pauli, G. F, Case, R. J, Inui, T, Wang, Y, Cho, S, Fischer, N. H, et al. New perspectives on natural products in TB drug research. Life Sci (2005). , 78(5), 485-94.

[48] Copp, B. R. Antimycobacterial natural products. Nat Prod Rep (2003). , 20(6), 535-57.

[49] Copp, B. R, & Pearce, A. N. Natural product growth inhibitors of Mycobacterium tu-
      berculosis. Nat Prod Rep (2007). , 24(2), 278-97.

[50] Guzman, J. D, et al. Antimycobacterials from natural sources: ancient times, antibiot-
      ic era and novel scaffolds. Front Biosci. (2012). , 17, 1861-81.

[51] Bueno-sanchez, J, Martínez-moralez, J, & Stashenko, E. a Actividad antimicobacteri-
      ana de terpenos. Salud UIS (2009). , 41-231.

[52] Bueno-sanchez, J, Martínez-moralez, J, Stashenko, E, & Ribón, W. b Anti-tubercular
      activity of eleven aromatic and medicinal plants occurring in Colombia. Biomédica.
      (2009). , 29-51.

[53] Baquero, E, Quiñones, W, Ribon, W, Caldas, M. L, Sarmiento, L, & Echeverri, F. Ef-
      fect of anoxadiazoline and a lignan on mycolic acid biosynthesis and ultrastructural
      changesof mycobacterium tuberculosis. Tuberculosis Research and Treatment.
      (2011).

[54] Guzman, J. D, Gupta, A, Evangelopoulos, D, Basavannacharya, C, Pabon, L. C, Pla-
      zas, E. A, Muñoz, D. R, Delgado, W. A, Cuca, L. E, Ribon, W, Gibbons, S, & Bhakta, S.
      Anti-tubercular screening of natural products from Colombian plants: 3-methoxy-
      nordomesticine, an inhibitor of MurE ligase of Mycobacterium tuberculosis.J Antimi-
      crobChemother. (2010). Oct;, 65(10), 2101-7.

[55] Ichiba, T, Corgiar, J. M, Scheuer, P. J, & Kelly-borges, M. 8-hydroxymanzamine A, a
      betacarboline alkaloid from a sponge, Pachypllina sp. J Nat Prod (1994). , 57(1),
      168-70.

[56] Yousaf, M, Hammond, N. L, Peng, J, Wahyuono, S, Mclntosh, K A, Charman, W N,
      Mayer, A M, & Hamann, M T. New manzamine alkaloids from a Indo-Pacific
      sponge. Pharmacokinetcs oral availability and the significant activity of several man-
      zaminesagainst HIV-I, AIDS opportunistic infections and inflammatory diseases. J
      MedChem. (2004). , 47(14), 3512-7.

[57] Davies, G. R, & Nuermberger, E. L. Pharmacokinetics and pharmacodynamics in the
      development of anti-tuberculosis drugs. Tuberculosis (2008). Suppl 1 S, 65-74.

[58] Matsuzaki, K. Why and how are peptide-lipid interactions utilized for self-defense?
      Magainins and tachyplesins as archetypes.BiochimBiophysActa (1999). A), J., Kratky,
      M. Development of new MDR-tuberculosis drugs. Nova Science Publishers, Inc; 2011

[59] Tripathi, R. P, Tewari, N, Dwivedi, N, & Tiwari, V. K. Fighting tuberculosis: and old-
      disease with new challenges. Med Res Rev (2005). , 25(1), 93-131.

[60] Barry, C, Cole, S, Fourie, B, Geiter, L, Gosey, L, & Grossey, J. et al. Scientific Blueprint
      forTuberculosis Drug Development, Published by the Global Alliance for TB Drug
      Development (2000). , 1-24.

[61] Lenaerts, A. J, Degroote, M. A, & Orme, I. M. Preclinical testing of new drugs for tuberculosis: current challenges. Trends Microbiol (2008). , 16(2), 48-54.

[62] Gehring, R, Schummb, P, Youssef, M, & Scoglio, C. A network-based approach for resistance transmission in bacterial populations. J Theor Biol. (2010). , 262(1), 97-106.

[63] Jayaram, R, Shandil, R. K, Gaonkar, S, Kaur, P, Suresh, B. L, Mahesh, B. N, et al. Isoniazidpharmacokinetics-pharmacodynamics in an aerosol infection model of tuberculosis.Antimicrob Agents Chemother.(2004). , 48(8), 2951-2957.

[64] Capuano, S. V, Croix, D. A, Pawar, S, Zinovik, A, Myers, A, Lin, P. L, et al. ExperimentalMycobacterium tuberculosis infection of cynomolgus macaques closely resemblesthe various manifestations of human M. tuberculosis infection. Infect Immun(2003). , 71(10), 5831-44.

[65] Janin, Y. L. Antituberculosis drugs: ten years of research. Bioorg Med Chem. (2007). , 15(7), 2479-513.

[66] Bogatcheva, E, Dubuisson, T, Protopopova, M, Einck, L, Nacy, C. A, & Reddy, V. M. Chemical modification of capuramycins to enhance antibacterial activity.J AntimicrobChemother (2011). , 66(3), 578-87.

[67] Cardona, P-J. editor. Understanding Tuberculosis- New Approaches to FightinAgainst Drug Resistance. Rijeka: InTech; (2012).

[68] Pasipanodya, . . A new evolutionary and pharmacokinetic-pharmacodynamics scenario for rapid emergence of resistance to single and multiple anti-tuberculosis drugs.CurrOpinPharmacol.2011;11(5)457-63.

[69] Barry, C, Cole, S, Fourie, B, & Geiter, L. Gosey, Grosset J, et al. Scientific Blueprint for TBDrug Development. The Global Alliance for TB Drug Development (2001). , 1-52.

[70] Brien, O. RJ. Studies of early bactericidal activity of new drugs for tuberculosis.Am. J.Resp. Crit. Care. Med. (2002). , 166(1), 3-4.

[71] Donald, P. R, & Diacon, A. H. The early bactericidal activity of anti-tuberculosis drugs: aliterature review, Tuberculosis (2008). Suppl 1 S, 75-83.

[72] Burman, W. J. The hunt for the elusive surrogate marker of sterilizing activity in tuberculosis treatment.Am J RespCrit Care Med (2003). , 167-1299.

[73] Mitchison, D. A. Clinical development of antituberculosis drugs. J AntimicrobChemother (2006). , 58(3), 494-95.

[74] The Global Alliance for TB Drug DevelopmentHandbook of anti-tuberculosisagents.TMC-207.Tuberculosis (2008). , 88(2), 168-69.

[75] Vinsova, J, & Kratky, M. Development of new MDR-tuberculosis drugs. Nova Science Publishers, Inc; (2011).

[76] The Global Alliance for TB Drug DevelopmentHandbook of anti-tuberculosis-agents.Gatifloxacin.Tuberculosis (2008). , 88(2), 109-11.

[77] The Global Alliance for TB Drug DevelopmentHandbook of anti-tuberculosis-agents.Moxifloxacin.Tuberculosis (2008). , 88(2), 127-31.

[78] The Global Alliance for TB Drug DevelopmentHandbook of anti-tuberculosis-agents.PA-824.Tuberculosis (2008). , 88(2), 134-36.

[79] Feuerriegel, S, Köser, C. U, Baù, D, Rüsch-gerdes, S, Summers, D. K, & Archer, J. A. Marti-Re-nom MA, Niemann S. Impact of Fgd1 and ddn diversity in Mycobacterium tuberculosis complex on in vitro susceptibility to PA-824. Antimicrob Agents Chemother(2011). , 55(12), 5718-22.

[80] The Global Alliance for TB Drug DevelopmentOPC-67683, Handbook of anti-tuberculosis agents. Tuberculosis (2008). , 88, 132-3.

[81] Nathan, C, Gold, B, Lin, G, Stegman, M, Carvalho, L. P, Vandal, O, Venugopal, A, & Bryk, R. A philosophy of anti-infectives as a guide in the search for new drugs for tuberculosis.Tuberculosis (Edinb). (2008). Suppl 1:S, 25-33.

[82] Festa, R. A, Pearce, M. J, & Darwin, K. H. Characterization of the proteasome accessory factor (paf) operon in Mycobacterium tuberculosis. J Bacteriol. (2007). , 189(8), 3044-50.

[83] Bashyam, H. Sabine Ehrt: searching for mycobacterial stress point. J Exp Med. (2008). , 205(10), 2184-2185.

[84] Boon, C, & Dick, T. How Mycobacterium tuberculosis goes to sleep: the dormancy survival regulator DosR a decade later. Future Microbiol (2012). , 7(4), 513-18.

[85] Mathuria, J. P. Nanoparticles in tuberculosis diagnosis, treatment and prevention: ahope for future. Digest Journal of Nanomaterials and Biostructures (2009). , 4(2), 309-12.

[86] Shegokar, R. Shaal LA Mitri K. ((2011). Present Status of Nanoparticle Research for-Treatment of Tuberculosis. J Pharm PharmSci 2011;, 14(1), 100-16.

Chapter 5

Web Resources on TB: Information, Research, and Data Analysis

Marcos Catanho and Antonio Basílio de Miranda

Additional information is available at the end of the chapter

1. Introduction

Since its creation in the middle of the 20th century, the Internet has become the universal language of the digital world. All the capabilities it offers, such as electronic mail systems, information distribution, file sharing, multimedia streaming services and online social networking, have already been of service to billions of people around the world. In fact, if the Internet were to disappear tomorrow, most people would struggle to manage their lives without it.

By providing millions of people with information that is constantly updated (24 hours a day, seven days a week) Internet has become the second source of information for the whole world, television still being the first one in most countries. It has also provided a unique way of communication, where a person in an isolated geographical location can instantly be in touch with thousands and maybe millions of other individuals around the world.

Scientists were among the first ones to explore all these capabilities. Now, we talk about data mining, terabytes and petabytes, algorithms – terms related to what we call "Big Data", the large volume of information generated by a variety of new technologies, ranging from Astronomy (telescope data), the Internet itself (more and more Facebook users every day) to Biology (cheaper and more efficient DNA sequencing technologies), among other areas of study and research. Some technologies and experiments, like the Large Hadron Collider at CERN, Switzerland (perhaps the most important scientific tool ever built), produce an incredible volume of information, on the order of terabytes per second.

Databases containing DNA and protein sequences were created; institutions around the world developed websites to expose their work to the world; scientific magazines started their online versions. The world is connected as never before. This connection transcend the virtual realm of the Internet: today, it is possible to travel from one side of the world to the other in just one day. Unfortunately, this has presented us a negative side: infectious agents may also cross the world in just about the same time.

Tuberculosis is a global disease, with an estimated one-third of all people in the world contaminated by the bacillus, *Mycobacterium tuberculosis*. Although treatable, the large period of treatment (many abandon the therapy as soon as they feel better) together with the indiscriminate use of antibiotics is causing the spread of new, drug-resistant strains. Actually, as those familiar with epidemiology have already noticed, that is a remarkable similarity between the patterns of an epidemic or outbreak with the spread of a new piece of information throughout the internet.

However, there has also been a revolution in other areas: new high-throughput technologies, like genomics, transcriptomics and proteomics, offer a new, more integrated view of the metabolism and genetics of the organism studied, and of course *M. tuberculosis* was among the first to have its genome sequenced. Today, more than 30 different strains have been sequenced, as well as other organisms from the *Mycobacterium* genus. By comparing the genomes of virulent and non-virulent strains of TB, scientists may pinpoint particular genes and/or polymorphisms involved in this process; by examining transcriptome data, researchers may have an idea of the effects of a given drug in the bacillus' metabolism.

The purpose of this chapter is by no means to offer an exhaustive list of all the resources available on the Internet about TB, the topic of this book. This would be a massive and perhaps futile work, since the evolution of the internet occurs at a very fast pace. Rather, this chapter concentrates on a selection of the most important, relevant and stable websites with relevance to several aspects of TB, such as research, treatment, main Institutions, funding, and specialized platforms. We think this should complement all the other information already presented in this book, offering the reader a more integrated view of the disease, and also access to new platforms and systems specialized in the analysis of data generated by a series of new technologies such as DNA sequencing.

2. Tuberculosis facts information and treatment research

Most of the selected sites presented in this section have information about several aspects of TB, like history, epidemiology, transmission and pathogenesis, diagnosis, treatment, infection control, besides offering other services such as courses, guidelines, fact sheets and links to related sites. We have chosen an alphabetical classification to avoid conveying a false impression of importance to some sites in detriment of others. In fact, we think that every effort is worthy in this global battle against this terrible disease.

Centers for Disease Control and Prevention. The mission of the Division of Tuberculosis Elimination (DTBE) is to promote health and quality of life by preventing, controlling, and eventually eliminating tuberculosis from the United States, and by collaborating with other countries and international partners in controlling global tuberculosis. URL: <http://www.cdc.gov/tb/>

Global Tuberculosis Institute. Located at the New Jersey Medical School, the institute provides expertise in program development, education, training and research to ministers of health, national TB programs and healthcare providers around the globe. URL: <http://www.umdnj.edu/globaltb/home.htm>

	Agency	URL
Americas	American Lung Association (ALA) Lung Disease Programs	http://www.lung.org/
	American Public Health Association	http://www.apha.org/
	Bill & Melinda Gates Foundation	http://www.gatesfoundation.org/
	CREATE: Consortium to Respond to the AIDS/TB Epidemic	http://www.tbhiv-create.org/
	Food and Drug Administration (FDA)	http://www.fda.gov/default.htm
	Institute for Tuberculosis Research	http://www.tuberculosisdrugresearch.org/
	National Institute of Allergy and Infectious Diseases (NIAID)	http://www.niaid.nih.gov/
	National Library of Medicine, PubMed	http://www.ncbi.nlm.nih.gov/entrez/query.fcgi
	Tuberculosis Net	http://tuberculosis.net/
Africa	AllAfrica.com: TB News from Africa	http://allafrica.com/tuberculosis/
	Desmond Tutu TB Centre	http://sun025.sun.ac.za/portal/page/portal/Health_Sciences/English/Centres/dttc
	South African Tuberculosis Vaccine Initiative	http://www.satvi.uct.ac.za/
Asia and Oceania	JATA - Research Institute of Tuberculosis	http://www.jata.or.jp/eindex/home.html
	National Institute for Research in Tuberculosis	http://www.trc-chennai.org/
	Pakistan Anti TB Association	http://www.patba.org/
	TBC India	http://www.tbcindia.nic.in/
Europe	European Tuberculosis Surveillance Network	http://www.ecdc.europa.eu/en/activities/surveillance/european_tuberculosis_surveillance_network/Pages/index.aspx
	International Union Against Tuberculosis and Lung Disease (UNION)	http://www.theunion.org/
	Max Planck Institute for Infection Biology	http://www.mpiib-berlin.mpg.de/
	Pasteur Institute	http://www.pasteur.fr

Table 1. Additional websites covering tuberculosis facts information and treatment research

Pan American Health Organization (PAHO). Serving as the regional office for WHO, PAHO has been working for more than one century to improve health and the living standards of the countries of the Americas, being recognized as part of the United Nations' system. URL: <http://new.paho.org/hq/>

StopTB Partnership. The StopTb Partnership operates through a secretariat hosted by the World Health Organization (WHO) in Geneva, Switzerland, and seven working groups whose role is to accelerate progress on access to TB diagnosis and treatment, research and development for new TB diagnostics, drugs and vaccines, and tackling drug resistant- and HIV-associated TB. URL: <http://www.stoptb.org/>

Tb Alliance. Established in the year 2000, its main objective is to discover and develop better, faster-acting, and affordable drugs to fight tuberculosis. Today, the organization and its partners manage a portfolio of new anti-Tb drugs. URL: <http://www.tballiance.org>

World Health Organization (WHO). Created in 1948, WHO is the directing and coordinating authority in international health within the United Nations' system, composed of 193 countries and two associate members. It supports and promotes health research in several areas, Tb being one of them. URL: <http://who.int/topics/tuberculosis/en/>

3. Tuberculosis databases and platforms

Since the emergence of Bioinformatics and Computational Biology back in the 1960's, numerous databases and computational tools have been created in order to provide the scientific community the necessary means to access and interpret a range of biological data.

Actually, the contribution of these disciplines became particularly evident in the 1990's and 2000's, when the development of supercomputers, powerful personal computers, and computer networks at global scale, as well as of high-throughput technologies, collectively referred as *omics* – *e.g.*, genomics, transcriptomics, and proteomics –, revolutionized the field of Biology.

Nowadays, a number of web resources are publicly available aiming to organize, integrate, and provide efficient access to the ever-increasing amount of biological information produced over decades of research, particularly in recent years, with numerous projects applying the aforementioned high-throughput technologies worldwide. Accordingly, diverse options to visualize, search, retrieve and analyze this wealth of data are offered, providing the opportunity to acquire more detailed knowledge about genomes and their respective organisms, among many others opportunities.

However, the creation and maintenance of such web resources is a challenge by itself, not only because they usually have to deal with large amounts of data, but mostly because they require the designing of schemes and frameworks that accurately represent the complexity of biological systems, which is frequently a hard task to be accomplished. Another difficulty is the development of efficient data retrieval systems, implemented in user-friendly interfaces and intended for complex and massive database searching. It is worth noting that, in many circumstances, the authors and curators of such resources receive little or no remuneration for their productive efforts, and the access to financial support for creation and maintenance of biological databases is still a difficult task.

In this section we present the main web resources fully or partially dedicated to mycobacterial species with relevance for readers interested in TB. Each database or platform, categorized according to its purpose and functionality, is quickly reviewed, and references to the original paper describing it, as well as its electronic site, are provided, serving as a guideline for researches or students working on TB. Notably, the computational resources presented here are all publicly available as online services and can potentially be applied to the identification of new drug targets, vaccine antigens, or diagnostics for TB, among many others applications.

3.1. Generic and multifunctional

MyBASE. The Mycobacterial Database [1] is an integrated platform for functional and evolutionary genomic study of the genus *Mycobacterium*, comprising extensive literature review and data annotation on mycobacterial genome polymorphism, virulence factors, and essential genes. URL: <http://mybase.psych.ac.cn/>

TBDB. The TB Database [2] provides a comprehensive genomic data repository for *M. tuberculosis* and related bacteria, combining (*in silico*) genome sequence and annotation data and (experimental) gene-expression data. It also provides an analysis platform with suitable computational tools to assist (comparative) genomic and gene-expression studies of these microorganisms. Annotated features of genes and genomes, predicted orthologous groups, operons and synteny blocks, as well as predicted and curated immunological epitopes and gene-expression patterns are available. URL: <http://www.tbdb.org/>

The MycoBrowser portal. The Mycobacterial Browser portal [3] is an extensive genomic and proteomic data repository for four related mycobacteria: *M. tuberculosis* H37Rv, *M. leprae* TN, *M. marinum* M, and *M. smegmatis* MC2. The system provides *in silico* generated and manually reviewed information on the complete genome sequence of these organisms. As part of this portal, the **TubercuList** database [4] integrates a range of information on the *M. tuberculosis* genome, such as genomic and protein annotations and features, drug and transcriptome data, mutant and operon annotation, and comparative genomics. It represents a complete redesign of the database with the same name provided by the GenoList genome browser (also described in this chapter). URL: <http://mycobrowser.epfl.ch/>

3.2. Genomic mapping and data mining

TubercuList, BoviList, BCGList. The GenoList [5] is a collection of databases dedicated to microbial genome analysis, providing a complete data set of protein and nucleotide sequences for selected species, as well as annotation and functional classification of these sequences. The TubercuList, BoviList, and BCGList databases are devoted to collect and integrate various aspects of the genomic information of *M. tuberculosis* H37Rv, *M. bovis* AF2122/97, and *M. bovis* BCG Pasteur 1173P2, respectively. URL: <http://genolist.pasteur.fr/>

TBrowse. The TBrowse [6] is a genomic data resource, based on the Generic Model Organism Database (a collection of open source computational tools for creating and managing genome-scale biological databases); the browse provides the scientific community an integrative genomic map of *M. tuberculosis* with millions of data-points representing different genomic features and computational predictions systematically collected from online resources and publications, including gene/operon predictions, orthologs, gene expression data, non-coding RNA, pathway/networks, regulatory elements, variation and repeats, subcellular localization, among others. URL: <http://tbrowse.osdd.net>

3.3. Comparative genomics

GenoMycDB. The GenoMycDB [7] is a relational database for large-scale comparative analysis of completely sequenced mycobacterial genomes based on their predicted protein content. Currently, the database comprises six mycobacteria – *M. tuberculosis* (strains H37Rv and CDC1551), *M. bovis* AF2122/97, *M. avium subsp. paratuberculosis* K10, *M. leprae* TN, and *M. smegmatis* MC2 155 – providing for each of their encoded protein sequences the predicted subcellular localization, the assigned cluster of orthologous groups (COGs), features of the corresponding gene, and links to several important databases; in addition, pairs or groups of homologs between selected species/strains can be dynamically inferred based on user-defined criteria. URL: <http://www.dbbm.fiocruz.br/GenoMycDB.html>

MycoDB. The xBASE [8] is another collection of databases, this one dedicated to bacterial comparative genome analyses. It provides precomputed data of comparative genome analyses among selected bacterial genera, as well as inferred orthologous groups and functional annotations. It also provides precomputed analyses of codon usage, base composition, codon adaptation index (CAI), hydropathy, and aromaticity of the protein coding sequences in these bacteria. As part of this multi-microbial system, the MycoDB currently comprises comparative data from 61 completely sequenced or unfinished mycobacterial genomes, including 40 strains of *M. tuberculosis*, *M. bovis* AF2122/97, *M. bovis* BCG strains Pasteur 1173P2 and Tokyo 172, among others mycobacteria. URL: <http://www.xbase.ac.uk/>

Mycobacterium tuberculosis Comparative Database. This Broad Institute's database comprises precomputed comparative genome analyses data of eight *M. tuberculosis* patient isolates with relevant clinical phenotypes and disease epidemiology (varied degree of spread, drug resistance, and clinical severity): *M. tuberculosis* F11, *M. tuberculosis* Haarlem, *M. tuberculosis* KZN 4207 (DS), *M. tuberculosis* KZN 1435 (MDR), *M. tuberculosis* KZN 605 (XDR), *M. tuberculosis* C, *M. tuberculosis* 98-R604 INH-RIF-EM, and *M. tuberculosis* W-148. Among the comparative data provided by this TB resource we can cite: inferred families of orthologous genes, genomic two-dimensional dot plot matrices, comparative genome mapping and browsing, and several comparative gene annotations and features. URL: <http://www.broadinstitute.org/annotation/genome/mycobacterium_tuberculosis_spp/MultiHome.html>

3.4. Genetic diversity and epidemiology

MGDD. The Mycobacterial Genome Divergence Database [9] comprises a data repository of genetic variations among different organisms belonging to the *M. tuberculosis* complex. The MGDD system provides quick searches for precomputed single nucleotide polymorphisms (SNPs), insertions/deletions, repeat expansions, and divergent sequences (inversions, duplications, and changes in synteny) in genomic regions of fully sequenced *M. tuberculosis* complex species and strains genomes. URL: <http://mirna.jnu.ac.in/mgdd/>

MIRU-VNTRplus. The Mycobacterial Interspersed Repetitive Unit – Variable Number Tandem Repeat (MIRU-VNTR) database [10,11] comprises a collection of 186 well characterized strains representing the major *M. tuberculosis* complex in which, for each strain, species, lineage, and epidemiologic information are provided together with 24 MIRU loci, Spoligotype patterns, Regions of Difference (RD) profiles, Single Nucleotide Polymorphisms (SNPs), susceptibility data, and IS6110 Restriction Fragment Length Polymorphism (RFLP) fingerprint images. The system enables users to analyze genotyping data of their own strains alone or in comparison with the reference strains in the database; analyses and comparisons of genotypes can be based on Multiple Locus VNTR Analysis (MLVA), Spoligotypes, Large Sequence Polymorphism (LSP) and SNPs data, or on a weighted combination of these markers. Tools for data analysis include: search for similar strains, creation of phylogenetic and minimum spanning trees and mapping of geographic information. URL: <http://www.miru-vntrplus.org>

MTCID. The *M. tuberculosis* Clinical Isolate Genetic Polymorphism Database [12] consists in a repository of genetic polymorphisms, providing Single Nucleotide Polymorphism (SNPs) and Spoligotype profiles of clinical isolates of *M. tuberculosis*, based on published literature and manual curation. URL: <http://ccbb.jnu.ac.in/Tb/>

SITVITWEB. The SITVITWEB [13] is a multi-marker database, comprising three major types of molecular markers: Spoligotypes, Mycobacterial Interspersed Repetitive Units (MIRUs) and Variable Number Tandem Repeat (VNTRs); this webserver is dedicated to the investigation of *M. tuberculosis* genetic diversity and molecular epidemiology. Currently, this international resource provides genotyping information on 62,582 *M. tuberculosis* complex clinical isolates from 153 countries of patient origin. URL: <http://www.pasteur-guadeloupe.fr:8081/SITVIT_ONLINE/>

Additionally, a few relevant computational tools are currently available as web services dedicated to analyze the genetic diversity of *M. tuberculosis* complex strains and characterize TB dynamics using molecular epidemiological data:

The **spolTools** [14] comprise a collection of browser programs designed to manipulate and analyze Spoligotype data of the *M. tuberculosis* complex, consisting in an online repository of Spoligotype isolates collected from various published data sets (currently, 1179 Spoligotypes and 6278 isolates across 30 datasets), and online tools for manipulating and analyzing these data (computation of basic population genetic quantities; visualization of clusters of Spoligotype patterns based on an estimated evolutionary history; and a procedure to predict emerging strains/genotypes associated with elevated transmission). URL: <http://www.emi.unsw.edu.au/spolTools/>

The **TB-Insight** [15] is a collection of computational methods (based on different models and datasets) for both lineage classification of *M. tuberculosis* complex strains, and for visualization of genetic diversity in *M. tuberculosis* complex population and distribution by lineage, as well as visual representation of associations between patient and strain groups, providing perception on differences in phenotypic characteristics, and phylogeographic associations of *M. tuberculosis* complex strains with host populations. URL: <http://tbinsight.cs.rpi.edu/>

3.5. Gene expression and regulation

MTBRegList. The MTBRegList [16] is dedicated to the analysis of gene expression and regulation data in *M. tuberculosis*, containing predicted and characterized regulatory motifs cross-referenced with their respective transcription factor(s), experimentally identified transcription start sites, and DNA binding sites. URL: <http://www.usherbrooke.ca/vers/MtbRegList>

MycoperonDB. The MycoperonDB [17] is a repository of known and computationally predicted operons and transcriptional units of (currently) five different mycobacteria – *M. tuberculosis* (strains H37Rv and CDC1551), *M. bovis* AF2122/97, *M. avium subsp. paratuberculosis* K10, and *M. leprae* TN – whose genomes have been completely sequenced. Presently, it comprises 18,053 genes organized as 8,256 predicted operons and transcriptional units, providing literature links for experimentally characterized operons, and access to known promoters and related information. URL: <http://cdfd.org.in/mycoperondb/home.html>

MTBreg. The MTBreg is part of the online services provided by the UCLA-DOE Institute for Genomics and Proteomics (http://www.doe-mbi.ucla.edu/), and consists in a repository of conditionally regulated proteins in *M. tuberculosis* grown under several different conditions mimicking infection; the database provides information on proteins that are regulated by selected transcription factors or other regulatory proteins, as well as on the experimental condition, the experimental dataset and a literature reference. URL: <http://www.doe-mbi.ucla.edu/Services/MTBreg/>

MycoRegDB. The Mycobacterial Promoter and Regulatory Elements Database [18] is part of a user-friendly web interface (**RegAnalyst**) that integrates a motif prediction program (MoPP), a pattern detection tool (MyPatternFinder), and a database of promoter and regulatory elements from various mycobacterial species (MycoRegDB). Currently, the MycoRegDB comprises the following species: *M. tuberculosis* (strains H37Rv and CDC1551), *M. bovis* BCG, *M. leprae*, *M. smegmatis*, *M. avium* subsp. *paratuberculosis*, *M. marinum*, *M. ulcerans*, *M. gilvum*, and *M. vanbaalenii*. For each database entry, a variety of useful information is provided, such as, gene annotation, CDS positions, promoter/regulatory sequence (with Transcription Start Point (TSP) or binding site explicitly marked), TSP-CDS/Motif-CDS distance, among others. The first release of MycoRegDB contained 290 annotated DNA motifs (174 promoters and 116 transcription factor binding sites) described in 81 research papers, according to the authors.. URL: <http://www.nii.ac.in/~deepak/RegAnalyst/MycoRegDB>

3.6. Structural biology

MtbSD. The *M. tuberculosis* Structural Database [19] is a resource dedicated to 3D protein structures of *M. tuberculosis*, providing relevant information on description, reaction catalyzed, domains, active sites, structural homologs and similarities between bound and cognate ligands. Currently, the database comprises 876 structures for 332 mycobacterial genes. URL: <http://bmi.icmr.org.in/mtbsd/MtbSD.php>

3.7. Drug targets and resistance

TDR Targets database. The Tropical Disease Research (TDR/WHO) Targets database [20] comprises extensive genetic, biochemical and pharmacological data related to tropical disease pathogens, including *M. tuberculosis*, as well as computationally predicted druggability for potential targets and compound desirability information; the goal is to exploit the availability of diverse datasets to facilitate the identification and prioritization of drugs and drug targets in neglected disease pathogens, such as the tubercle bacillus. URL: <http://tdrtargets.org/>

TB Drug Resistance Mutation Database. The Tuberculosis Drug Resistance Mutation Database [21] is a comprehensive database that catalogs mutations associated with TB drug resistance and the frequency of the most common mutations associated with resistance to specific drugs, providing a resource for the development of molecular diagnostics for TB, as well as structural mapping of mutations to investigate mechanisms of resistance for drug discovery purposes. URL: <http://www.tbdreamdb.com/>

4. Conclusion

As outlined in this chapter, Informatics has acquired a great importance not only in the biological sciences, but in all areas of knowledge. Internet has become one of the most important tools for most people, from a dedicated researcher interested in the latest advances in his/her particular field of work to the teenager trying to contact his friends. Companies, industries and research institutes developed sites, where they expose their work to laymen.

The large number of publicly available databases and computational tools that have been developed, dedicated to organize, integrate, and provide efficient access to the ever-increasing amount of biological information produced over decades of research, have benefited researchers all over the world, especially those from low-income countries.

One important drawback, that still has to be overcome, is that the wealth of biological information available is presently fragmented, dispersed across numerous computational resources, and is redundant in many circumstances, clearly requiring unification in order to provide a global and integral picture of the biological systems they are dedicated to.

Ideally, the upcoming databases and computational tools should offer: data integration, providing multi-perspective analyses; combine *in silico* generated and manually curated data, improving the quality of our research; present efficient data structure, storage and processing, providing dynamic, flexible and fast data visualization, data searching, data retrieval and data analysis, via user-friendly graphical interfaces; implement a consistent and controlled vocabulary to describe the data and standardized data formats, providing full data inter-changing and integration with other data sources. We believe that only in this way, a fruitful field for interactions and cooperation among researches from distinct areas might emerge, providing the required support to interpret and analyze this wealth of data according to a truly multidisciplinary approach.

Author details

Marcos Catanho[1*] and Antonio Basílio de Miranda[2]

*Address all correspondence to: mcatanho@fiocruz.br

1 Laboratory for Functional Genomics and Bioinformatics, Oswaldo Cruz Institute, Rio de Janeiro, Brazil

2 Laboratory of Computational Biology and Systems, Oswaldo Cruz Institute, Rio de Janeiro, Brazil

References

[1] Zhu, X, Chang, S, Fang, K, Cui, S, Liu, J, Wu, Z, et al. MyBASE: a database for ge-nome polymorphism and gene function studies of Mycobacterium. BMC Microbiol (2009).

[2] Reddy, T. B, Riley, R, Wymore, F, Montgomery, P, Decaprio, D, Engels, R, et al. TB database: an integrated platform for tuberculosis research. Nucleic Acids Res (2009). Jan;37(Database (D499-D508)

[3] Kapopoulou, A, Lew, J. M, & Cole, S. T. The MycoBrowser portal: a comprehensive and manually annotated resource for mycobacterial genomes. Tuberculosis (Edinb) (2011). Jan;, 91(1), 8-13.

[4] Lew, J. M, Kapopoulou, A, Jones, L. M, & Cole, S. T. TubercuList--10 years after. Tu-berculosis (Edinb) (2011). Jan;, 91(1), 1-7.

[5] Lechat, P, Hummel, L, Rousseau, S, & Moszer, I. GenoList: an integrated environ-ment for comparative analysis of microbial genomes. Nucleic Acids Res (2008). Jan; 36(Database (D469-D474)

[6] Bhardwaj, A, Bhartiya, D, Kumar, N, & Scaria, V. TBrowse: an integrative genomics map of Mycobacterium tuberculosis. Tuberculosis (Edinb) (2009). Sep;, 89(5), 386-7.

[7]   Catanho, M, Mascarenhas, D, Degrave, W, & Miranda, A. B. GenoMycDB: a database for comparative analysis of mycobacterial genes and genomes. Genet Mol Res (2006). Mar 31;, 5(1), 115-26.

[8]   Chaudhuri, R. R, Loman, N. J, Snyder, L. A, Bailey, C. M, Stekel, D. J, & Pallen, M. J. xBASE2: a comprehensive resource for comparative bacterial genomics. Nucleic Acids Res (2008). Jan;36(Database (D543-D546)

[9]   Vishnoi, A, Srivastava, A, Roy, R, & Bhattacharya, A. MGDD: Mycobacterium tuberculosis genome divergence database. BMC Genomics (2008).

[10] Allix-beguec, C, Harmsen, D, Weniger, T, Supply, P, & Niemann, S. Evaluation and strategy for use of MIRU-VNTRplus, a multifunctional database for online analysis of genotyping data and phylogenetic identification of Mycobacterium tuberculosis complex isolates. J Clin Microbiol (2008). Aug;, 46(8), 2692-9.

[11] Weniger, T, Krawczyk, J, Supply, P, Niemann, S, & Harmsen, D. MIRU-VNTRplus: a web tool for polyphasic genotyping of Mycobacterium tuberculosis complex bacteria. Nucleic Acids Res (2010). Jul;38(Web Server (W326-W331)

[12] Bharti, R, Das, R, Sharma, P, Katoch, K, & Bhattacharya, A. MTCID: a database of genetic polymorphisms in clinical isolates of Mycobacterium tuberculosis. Tuberculosis (Edinb) (2012). Mar;, 92(2), 166-72.

[13] Demay, C, Liens, B, Burguiere, T, Hill, V, Couvin, D, Millet, J, et al. SITVITWEB--a publicly available international multimarker database for studying Mycobacterium tuberculosis genetic diversity and molecular epidemiology. Infect Genet Evol (2012). Jun;, 12(4), 755-66.

[14] Tang, C, Reyes, J. F, Luciani, F, Francis, A. R, & Tanaka, M. M. spolTools: online utilities for analyzing spoligotypes of the Mycobacterium tuberculosis complex. Bioinformatics (2008). Oct 15;, 24(20), 2414-5.

[15] Shabbeer, A, Ozcaglar, C, Yener, B, & Bennett, K. P. Web tools for molecular epidemiology of tuberculosis. Infect Genet Evol (2012). Jun;, 12(4), 767-81.

[16] Jacques, P. E, Gervais, A. L, Cantin, M, Lucier, J. F, Dallaire, G, Drouin, G, et al. MtbRegList, a database dedicated to the analysis of transcriptional regulation in Mycobacterium tuberculosis. Bioinformatics (2005). May 15;, 21(10), 2563-5.

[17] Ranjan, S, Gundu, RK, Ranjan, A, & Mycoperon, . : a database of computationally identified operons and transcriptional units in Mycobacteria. BMC Bioinformatics 2006;7 Suppl 5:S9.

[18] Sharma, D, Mohanty, D, & Surolia, A. RegAnalyst: a web interface for the analysis of regulatory motifs, networks and pathways. Nucleic Acids Res (2009). Jul;37(Web Server (W193-W201)

[19] Hassan, S, Logambiga, P, Raman, AM, Subazini, TK, Kumaraswami, V, Hanna, LE, &
      Mtb, . --a comprehensive structural database for Mycobacterium tuberculosis. Tuber-
      culosis (Edinb) 2011 Nov;91(6):556-62.

[20] Aguero, F, Al-lazikani, B, Aslett, M, Berriman, M, Buckner, F. S, Campbell, R. K, et al.
      Genomic-scale prioritization of drug targets: the TDR Targets database. Nat Rev
      Drug Discov (2008). Nov;, 7(11), 900-7.

[21] Sandgren, A, Strong, M, Muthukrishnan, P, Weiner, B. K, Church, G. M, & Murray,
      M. B. Tuberculosis drug resistance mutation database. PLoS Med (2009). Feb
      10;6(2):e2.

Chapter 6

Economic Evaluation of Diagnosis Tuberculosis in Hospital Setting

Luciene C. Scherer

Additional information is available at the end of the chapter

1. Introduction

Tuberculosis (TB) is an ancient disease, but not a disease of the past. After disappearing from the world public health agenda in the 1960s and 1970s, TB returned in the early 1990s for several reasons, including the emergence of the HIV/AIDS pandemic and the increase in drug resistance. More than 100 years after the discovery of the tubercle bacillus by Robert Koch, what is the status of TB control worldwide? The evolution of global TB control policies, including DOTS (Directly Observed Therapy, Short course) and the Stop TB Strategy, and assess whether the challenges and obstacles faced by the public health community worldwide in developing and implementing this strategy can aid future action towards the elimination of TB.(Lienhardt, Glaziou et al. 2012) The report of the Commission on Macroeconomics and Health of the World Health Organization has emphasized that tuberculosis is the most common of the infectious diseases. Tuberculosis is one of the most important health problems in the world, causing 1.4 million deaths each year, in 2011. (WHO, 2010)

The most of TB cases (82%) was concentrated in 22 countries around the world. In the year of 2010, in Brazil were detected 81946 cases, with 5000 death (WHO, 2010).

In Rio Grande do Sul, a state in extreme south of Brazil, the incidence of TB in 2011 was 46,1 per 100.000, with 4947 new cases. Porto Alegre, capital of Rio Grande do Sul shows incidence of 116 in 2009.(Sul 2011; Brazil 2012)

Tuberculosis is the first cause of death in patients with AIDS in Brazil. Patients with co-infection HIV/TB have had in treatment of Tuberculosis probability of worst outcome.

Rio Grande do Sul, has had the major incidence of TB/HIV co-infection. The co-infection adversely affects the lives of individuals in both the biological and psychosocial aspects. (Neves, Canini et al. 2012)

Some factors can be considered as risk factors for co-infection of TB and HIV, as the impoverishment of the population, use of injecting drugs, the disruption of services on the epidemiology of TB control, the delay in the diagnosis of TB and increased risk of acquiring multi-drug resistant TB (MDRTB), essentially associated to the expansion of the disease in the world.(Kritski, Lapa e Silva et al. 1998). Multidrug-resistant tuberculosis (MDR-TB) is a major clinical challenge, particularly in patients with human immunodeficiency virus (HIV) co-infection.(Nathanson, Nunn et al. ; Farley, Ram et al. 2011; Arjomandzadegan, Titov et al. 2012; Jain, Dixit et al. 2012; Udwadia 2012)

For the above, in recent years became consensus that the epidemic of TB in developing countries demands the evaluation of broader approaches, described in the Plan STOP-TB/OMS control global TB 2006-2015.

Among them have been prioritizing the implementation of:

a) improvements in access to diagnostic system user health; b) culture for mycobacteria in every patient suspected of TB and HIV positive and all TB patients in retreatment; c) sensitivity test for suspected cases of resistant TB (retreatment cases, treatment failure, contact MDR-TB or have been treated at the Health Unit with a high rate TB-MDR/XDR); d) review and economic evaluation under routine conditions of deployment of new technologies (phenotypic or molecular, automated or not) for the early diagnosis of TB, resistant TB patients with paucibacillary TB, HIV-infected or suspected drug-resistant TB.

Early detection of tuberculosis (TB) is essential for infection control. Rapid clinical diagnosis is more challenging in patients who have co-morbidities, such as Human Immunodeficiency Virus (HIV) infection. Direct microscopy has low sensitivity and culture takes 3 to 6 weeks (Sharma, Mohan et al. 2005; WHO 2006). Diagnostic testing for tuberculosis has remained unchanged for nearly a century, but newer technologies hold promise for a revolution in tuberculosis diagnostics. Tests such as the nucleic acid amplification assays commercial and in house technologies allow more rapid and accurate diagnosis of pulmonary and extrapulmonary tuberculosis.(Rodrigues Vde, Queiroz Mello et al. 2002; Sanchez, Rossetti et al. 2006; Scherer, Sperhacke et al. 2007; Scherer, Sperhacke et al. 2011; Hida, Hisada et al. 2012). Xpert MTB/RIF (Xpert) is actually a promising new rapid diagnostic technology for tuberculosis (TB) which has characteristics that suggests large-scale roll-out.(Vassall, van Kampen et al. 2011). In developing countries, *in house* Polymerase Rhain reaction (PCR) based on amplifying the IS6110 insertion element can be used for the amplification of *Mycobacterium tuberculosis* (MTB) DNA and offers the potential of a sensitive, specific and rapid diagnostic for ruling out or considering pulmonary tuberculosis (PTB) (Mehrotra, Metz et al. 2002; Sarmiento, Weigle et al. 2003; Schijman, Losso et al. 2004; Flores, Pai et al. 2005).

The appropriate and affordable use of any of these tests depends on the setting in which they are employed (Perkins 2000; Brodie and Schluger 2005). New tools for TB diagnosis, treatment and control are necessary, especially in health settings with a high prevalence of HIV/TB co-infection.

Although TB is one the greatest causes of mortality worldwide, its economic effects are not well known, especially in Brazil. Despite the fact that the families did not have to pay for medications and treatment, given that this service is offered by the State, the costs to families related to loss of income due to the disease were very high. The proportion of public service funds utilized for prevention is small. Greater investment in prevention campaigns not only might diminish the numbers of cases but also might lead to earlier diagnosis, thus reducing the costs associated with hospitalization. The lack of an integrated cost accounting system makes it impossible to visualize costs across the various sectors.(Costa, Santos et al. 2005)

To make rational decisions about the implementation of new tools in the medical routine, cost-effectiveness studies are essential(Mitarai, Kurashima et al. 2001; Kivihya-Ndugga, van Cleeff et al. 2003; Hazbon 2004).

A key step in cost-effectiveness analysis is to identify and value cost. The economic concept of opportunity cost is central to cost-effectiveness analysis. When a public health agency spends money to provide health care, this money is not available for housing, education, highway construction, or as a reduction in income taxes. When a health care organization spends money for bone transplantation, this money is not available for example for mammography outreach or something. When an elderly man spends time being vaccinated for influenza, this time is not available to play golf or to work. An overall conceptual goal in cost-effectiveness analysis is comprehensive identification of all costs of the intervention and its alternative, including all of the opportunity costs.

Contributors to cost must be identified before the costs can be valued. The terms used to describe the contributors to cost (e.g. direct costs, indirected costs, opportunity costs) are used in different ways in different textbooks and in published cost-effectiveness analysis.

The definition of cost terms is the opportunity cost is the value of resources in an alternative use, the direct cost is the value of all goods, services, and other resources consumed in the provision of an intervation or in dealing with the side effects or other current and future consequence linked to it and the productivity costs are the costs associated with lost or impaired ability to work or engage in leisure activities and lost economic productivity due to death attributable to the disease. These costs have been substituted for indirect costs. There are several categories of direct costs. The first category of total direct cost is direct health cost, this category include costs with tests, drugs, supplies, personnel, equipment, rent, depreciation, utilities, maintenance and support services. The second category of total direct cost is direct non- health care cost, these cost include for example the cost to patients to partake of the intervention e.g., transportation, child care, parking). The third category of total direct cost is the cost of informal caregiver time, this is the monetary value of the time of family members or volunteers who provide home care. The fourth category of total direct cost is the cost is the cost of the use of patient time. Such studies provide insight into the composition of different cost components, which may be the most important factor from the patient and the health service's perspectives. Recent studies have compared the cost effectiveness of news tools for diagnosis, treatment and control in Tuberculosis.(Amicosante, Ciccozzi et al. ; Kowada, Deshpande et al. ; Baltussen, Floyd et al. 2005; Barbieri, Wong et al. 2005; Bachmann 2006; Dwolatzky, Trengove et al. 2006; Kominski, Varon et al. 2007; Kowada,

Takahashi et al. 2008; Rosen, Taylor et al. 2010; Shi, Hodges et al. 2010; Vassall, van Kampen et al. 2011; Fitzpatrick and Floyd 2012; Lienhardt, Raviglione et al. 2012; Mandalakas, Hesseling et al. 2012). In a recent study we compared the cost-effectiveness of direct microscopy by Ziehl Neelsen staining (AFB smear) with *in house* polymerase chain reaction (PCR) and with culture on the first sputum specimen collection, including staff costs, using culture and clinical evaluation as the gold standard (Scherer, Sperhacke et al. 2009). In contrast to the cost-effectiveness analysis described by van Cleef et al. in a reference ambulatory clinic in Kenya, where only culture for mycobacteria was used as the gold standard (Roos, van Cleeff et al. 1998; van Cleeff, Kivihya-Ndugga et al. 2005). The cost-effectiveness of the AFB smear plus PCR dot-blot strategy described in recent study was similar to other strategies, when lower TB prevalence made PCR more expensive for diagnosis of PTB (Roos, van Cleeff et al. 1998; van Cleeff, Kivihya-Ndugga et al. 2005). (Scherer et. aL., 2009).

The mathematical models may be particularly useful for predicting the long term tendency of occurrence of the infection or disease. These models can simulate situations epidemiological and preventive or curative interventions beyond their theoretical impact in reducing the problem. Such predictive models properly formulated and fed with consistent data, may assist the processes of planning and management in public health. Currently several strategies have allowed the use of Multiple Logistic Regression (MLR) in the construction of predictive models. Models of decisions trees are also used for classification decision making or to provide a decision algorithm for the clinical management of infectious diseases.(Aguiar, Almeida et al. 2012)

For developing countries, the emergence of continuous technological innovation represents a double burden. The rapid diffusion of scientific and technical information that are observed now and monetary action multinational companies create a local demand for innovation by health professionals, the media and more informed portions of the population, which further strains the health care system.

Many factors limit the realization of a health technology assessment (HTA) analysis, as the lack of human resources, infrastructure or budget or due to lack of evidence or information costs.

Another obvious problem is that often decisions are based on scientific evidence coming from developed countries and often in settings where the incidence of disease differs effusively of Brazilian and Latin American scenario.

Given this scenario health managers are often between two objectives: they have to incorporate new and more costly technologies to improve the health of the population and at the same time are responsible for the financial sustainability and access equity of this in the system health.(Project 2005)

Beyond the suffering caused directly by the disease, TB is requiring significant portions of the public budget in developing countries. It is estimated that by 2015 they will be required investments around $12 billion for control of diseases such as AIDS, TB and Malaria. The increased costs involved in care and control of TB are due also to the increasing number of cases of resistant bacteria to different types of chemotherapy. (Polansky, Dymer et al. 1968; Garcia Rodriguez, Marino Callejo et al. 1994; Weis, Foresman et al. 1999; Gomes, Soares et al. 2003; Elamin, Ibrahim et al. 2008; Kik, Olthof et al. 2009; Steffen, Menzies et al. 2010; Vassall, Seme et al. 2010; Pereira, Barreto et al. 2012)

Costs of TB diagnosis and treatment may represent a significant burden for the poor and for the health system in resource-poor countries. Costs incurred by TB patients are high in Rio de Janeiro, especially for those under DOT. The DOT strategy doubles patients' costs and increases by fourfold the health system costs per completed treatment. The additional costs for DOT may be one of the contributing factors to the completion rates below the targeted 85% recommended by WHO (Steffen, Menzies et al. 2010).

Even in a country with a good health insurance system that covers medication and consultation costs, patients do have substantial extra expenditures. Furthermore, our patients lost on average 2.7 months of productive days. TB patients are economically vulnerable. (Kik, Olthof et al. 2009)

In Brazil, the real costs of TB are estimated or poorly known and the overall costs of TB are not perceived by governments, given the fragmentation in the involvement of the three governmental levels: local, state and national.

The purpose of this chapter is to describe the direct and indirect costs for diagnosis and treatment of Pulmonary Tuberculosis in patients infected or not by HIV, admitted to a Hospital Unit of Public Health.

2. Costs of health system of Brazil

In order to describe the costs of Health system of Brazil, we evaluate the costs directs of diagnosis and treatment of screening of 1000 hypothetical patients suspects of Pulmonary Tuberculosis in according with clinical and laboratory Brazilian recommendations for treatment (Tuberculose 2004; Conde, Melo et al. 2009).

The cost components for each clinical and laboratory procedures of screening included costs incurred by the patient, laboratory costs, drugs, consumables and equipment costs. The strategy for screening was the same recommended for Brazilian Public Health System.

Clinical, radiological and laboratory staff costs were calculated from the salary base of Rio Grande do Sul (State of Extreme South of Brazi) in 2011.

For each procedure, costs were attributed based on procedure costs of the Brazilian Public Health System.

Running costs (material costs were used for each 1000 tests evaluated) included all laboratory materials used in procedures.

All costs were expressed in US$, using an exchange rate of US$ 1= R$ 1,72 (REAIS), the average exchange rate from 2010 to 2011. In the treatment costs, those were evaluated related to the treatment of inpatients and outpatients. To estimate the values that are spent by the public health system of Brazil with the monitoring and control of TB in a hospital and an outpatient unit, we simulated two different scenarios:

a. TB cases diagnosed in hospital wards (hospitalized patients)

b. TB cases diagnosed in outpatient environment (outpatients).

The number of days considered to calculate the costs related to the treatment of inpatients they were considered as the same days that were spent in laboratory procedure.

It was hypothesized that the time to detect *Mycobacterium tuberculosis* in sputum culture from patients with pulmonary tuberculosis may be a better indicator for the duration of time of hospitalization(Ritchie, Harrison et al. 2007).

The time to detect *M. tuberculosis* in the culture was 30 days in this study. This cohort is the same as previous published by our group [20]. This value was used as the standard at which release from isolation could be permitted (Scherer, Sperhacke et al. 2007)

The time spent on laboratory procedure to provide access to the result of the laboratory technique was assumed to be 30 days for AFB smear plus culture. The number of days considered to calculate costs was the same as those spent on laboratory procedure. The number of days considered to calculate the cost of patient travel costs was assumed to be 2 days for AFB smear plus culture.

Total treatment included clinical officer and hospital costs, assuming cost per pill, to be US$ 0.22, using 3 pills per day, during 180 days; hospital room costs, US$ 7/day; costs with salary of clinical staff and clinical consultation, US$ 2.52 per patient and clinical nursing consultation, US$ 2.52 per patient.

Assuming that, during the treatment (6 months), in ambulatory situation, 6 AFB smear test, 6 chest radiographs, 6 consult of nurse and 2 consult of clinical were performed, we used this parameters to estimate the costs of ambulatory following the Brazilian recommendations for treatment (Tuberculose 2004).

Assuming that, during the hospitalization (30 days), 4 AFB smear tests, 4 chest radiographs, 30 nurse and physician consultations were performed, we used these parameters to estimate the costs of inpatient assistance in hospital, following the Brazilian recommendations for treatment (Tuberculose 2004; Conde, Melo et al. 2009). Staff salaries for the physician, nurse and radiologist were considered to be US$ 11,163 per year, and for the chest radiograph technician, the salary was US$ 4,988 per year. The work days were considered 20 days for all staff.

The days of admission to the hospital were considered to be the same number of days spent on each laboratory procedure. All estimated costs reflect an estimative of the public health system of Brazil expenses with the monitoring and control of TB.

The costs were expressed per 1000 suspects, according to the specific bibliographic references for economic analyses, thus, allowing the best decision for investment to be made (Petitti 2000).

Table 1A shows the costs at the health service level and Table 1B shows costs due to laboratory investment. The AFB smear plus Culture require (US$ 39,535) for equipment. Table 1C shows costs incurred by patients.

A. Health service costs

	Staff Number	Salaries of all staff per year (US$)	Staff Cost per day (US$)	Time spent until access to result (days)
AFB smear plus Culture	2	16,151	67	30

B. Laboratory costs

	Equipment (US$)	Annualization Years	Running costs per 1000 suspects (US$)	Running costs per examination (US$)
AFB smear plus Culturea	39,535	5	12,507	12.50

C. Estimated costs incurred by patients, including costs for travel, food and income loss[d]

	AFB smear plus Culture (US$) (outpatients and inpatients)
Travel	1,390
Food	10,000
Income Loss[c]	310,000
Total patients Cost	341,000

[a] Microscopic and Laminar Flow Cabinets. Other equipments were not included

[b] Income loss of patients was calculated from monthly salary base of Brazil (US$207) and was based on proportional days spent by patients until access to the result of each laboratory procedure. Patient costs were estimated using the average of two visits to the laboratory for AFB smear and culture procedures for outpatients; Travel cost was considered as US$ 1.4 (one bus ticket). Food was considered as US$ 10 per meal. Base salary in Brazil was considered (US$ 10 per day /20 days of the work). For inpatients was considered just income loss; Staff costs in the laboratory were based on proportional days spent on each laboratory procedure; Costs of consumables and equipment were provided by the program as well as by the manufacturer.

Table 1. Estimative of Costs in US$ in Tuberculosis Diagnosis in Brazil

We annualized the capital cost of the equipment for 5 years, according to the literature [25]. Building costs were not included. Opportunity costs were not applicable.

	AFB smear plus Culture
Laboratory Costs	
Labor Costs[a]	3,743
Investment costs	37
Running costs	3,700
Staff Costs per day	
Cost laboratory staff [b]	1,434
Cost of staff related to the treatment of patients[b]	2,791
Costs of chest radiograph staff related to the treatment of patients	404
Treatment Costs per day	
Costs of diagnostic service related to the treatment of no-hospitalized patients	2,771
Costs of diagnostic service related to the treatment of hospitalized patients	4,686
Treatment costs (hospitalized patients plus no- hospitalized patients)[c]	7,456
Income Loss	190,000
Total Patient costs	190,000
Total Health Service costs	9,479,033
Total Screening costs	9,668,815

[a] For each procedure, costs were attributed based on procedure costs of the Brazilian Public Health System (US$ 1,4 for AFB smear and US$ 1,9 for Culture) and from CDCT/FEPPS (US$ 11,7 for PCR dot-blot), assuming investment laboratory equipment for 5 years; [b]Staff salary was considered; for laboratory technician, US$2,860 per year; for Laboratory technologist, US$6,400 per year. Staff costs in the laboratory were based on proportional days spent on each laboratory procedure; Staff salary was considered for clinical physician, nurse and radiologist; US$6,400 per year; for the X-RAY technician, salary was US$2,860 per year. [c]The days of admission to the hospital were considered as the same as the days spent on each laboratory procedure. The time spent on each laboratory procedure until access to the result of the laboratory technique was assumed to be 30 days for AFB smear plus Culture. Total treatment included clinical officer and hospital costs, assuming US$ 0,22 cost per pill, using 3 pills for day, during 180 days; hospital room costs, US$ 4,16/day; costs of salary of staff clinical; clinical consultation cost, US$2,52 per patient; clinical nursing consultation, US $2,52 per patient. Assuming that during the treatment of inpatients (4 months) 4 ZN and 4 chest radiograph were performed, and during the treatment of no- hospitalized patients (6 months) 6 AFB smear and 6 chest radiograph were performed, following the Brazilian recommendations for treatment (Tuberculose 2004);

[d] Travel was considered 2 days for AFB smear plus Culture strategy. Food and income loss for AFB smear plus Culture strategy was considered 30 days

The health service costs analysis was based on processing 50 AFB smear slides and 14 cultures per day. AFB smear plus Culture was performed by two trained staff.

Running costs were calculated from investments required to examine 1000 smears.

Table 2. Total cost of screening for 1000 suspects. The total screening costs to AFB smear plus Culture were US$ 9,668.815.

The total cost (in US$) related to the treatment (no hospitalized patients) for AFB smear plus Culture was US$ 2,771. The cost related to the treatment of hospitalized patients, for AFB smear plus Culture strategy was US$ 4,686. The cost related to the treatment of (no hospitalized patients) and (hospitalized patients), for AFB smear plus Culture strategy was US$ 7,456.

However, in a context of advanced technologies for the diagnosis of tuberculosis, economic resources has always limited the incorporation and diffusion of new technologies produced and validated by the academy. It is a challenge for health systems worldwide, and in many cases, the cause of serious sustainability problems.(Taylor, Drummond et al. 2004; King, Griffin et al. 2006; Mason, Weatherly et al. 2007; Hughes, Tilson et al. 2009; Weatherly, Drummond et al. 2009; Shi, Hodges et al. 2010)

The decisions related to incorporation, acquisition, reimbursement or coverage of new technologies and those that determine the way in which they should be used are the most important in the health system and should be taken in general and the management of health services in particular.(Greenberg, Peterburg et al. 2005)

The health systems of different countries are diverse with respect to decisions about incorporating technologies and expectations of service users. Tough choices are faced by managers at all levels of the health system. This reality makes the TB every year, become more difficult for the system to provide the user with the most effective intervention theoretically available, depending on the pressures placed on the health system in relation to increased costs, the training of human resources, needs updating certification and regulatory instruments, and investment in physical infrastructure (Newhouse 1992)

Attempts to improve the acceptability of resource allocation decisions around new health technologies have spanned many years, fields and disciplines. Various theories of decision making have been tested and methods piloted, but, despite their availability, evidence of sustained uptake is limited. Since the challenge of determining which of many technologies to fund is one that healthcare systems have faced since their inception, an analysis of actual processes, criticisms confronted and approaches used to manage them may serve to guide the development of an 'evidence-informed' decision-making framework for improving the acceptability of decisions.(Stafinski, Menon et al. 2011)

Author details

Luciene C. Scherer

Lutheran University of Brasil-ULBRA, Canoas/ RS/, Brazil

References

[1] WHO (2010). "Global tuberculosis control: key findings from the December 2009 WHO report." Wkly Epidemiol Rec 85(9): 69-80.

[2] (2010). "WHO global tuberculosis control report 2010. Summary." Cent Eur J Public Health 18(4): 237.

[3] Aguiar, F. S., L. L. Almeida, et al. (2012). "Classification and regression tree (CART) model to predict pulmonary tuberculosis in hospitalized patients." BMC Pulm Med 12(1): 40.

[4] Amicosante, M., M. Ciccozzi, et al. "Rational use of immunodiagnostic tools for tuberculosis infection: guidelines and cost effectiveness studies." New Microbiol 33(2): 93-107.

[5] Arjomandzadegan, M., L. P. Titov, et al. (2012). "Determination of principal genotypic groups among susceptible, MDR and XDR clinical isolates of Mycobacterium tuberculosis in Belarus and Iran." Tuberk Toraks 60(2): 153-159.

[6] Bachmann, M. O. (2006). "Effectiveness and cost effectiveness of early and late prevention of HIV/AIDS progression with antiretrovirals or antibiotics in Southern African adults." AIDS Care 18(2): 109-120.

[7] Baltussen, R., K. Floyd, et al. (2005). "Cost effectiveness analysis of strategies for tuberculosis control in developing countries." BMJ 331(7529): 1364.

[8] Barbieri, M., J. B. Wong, et al. (2005). "The cost effectiveness of infliximab for severe treatment-resistant rheumatoid arthritis in the UK." Pharmacoeconomics 23(6): 607-618.

[9] Brazil (2012). "Ministry of Health-Epidemiological Report- Tuberculosis 2011."

[10] Brodie, D. and N. W. Schluger (2005). "The diagnosis of tuberculosis." Clin Chest Med 26(2): 247-271, vi.

[11] Conde, M. B., F. A. Melo, et al. (2009). "III Brazilian Thoracic Association Guidelines on tuberculosis." J Bras Pneumol 35(10): 1018-1048.

[12] Costa, J. G., A. C. Santos, et al. (2005). "[Tuberculosis in Salvador, Brazil: costs to health system and families]." Rev Saude Publica 39(1): 122-128.

[13] Dwolatzky, B., E. Trengove, et al. (2006). "Linking the global positioning system (GPS) to a personal digital assistant (PDA) to support tuberculosis control in South Africa: a pilot study." Int J Health Geogr 5: 34.

[14] Elamin, E. I., M. I. Ibrahim, et al. (2008). "Cost of illness of tuberculosis in Penang, Malaysia." Pharm World Sci 30(3): 281-286.

[15] Farley, J. E., M. Ram, et al. (2011). "Outcomes of multi-drug resistant tuberculosis (MDR-TB) among a cohort of South African patients with high HIV prevalence." PLoS One 6(7): e20436.

[16] Fitzpatrick, C. and K. Floyd (2012). "A systematic review of the cost and cost effectiveness of treatment for multidrug-resistant tuberculosis." Pharmacoeconomics 30(1): 63-80.

[17] Flores, L. L., M. Pai, et al. (2005). "In-house nucleic acid amplification tests for the detection of Mycobacterium tuberculosis in sputum specimens: meta-analysis and meta-regression." BMC Microbiol 5: 55.

[18] Garcia Rodriguez, J. F., A. Marino Callejo, et al. (1994). "[Hospital costs of tuberculosis]." Med Clin (Barc) 102(15): 596-597.

[19] Gomes, C., S. Soares, et al. (2003). "[The cost of tuberculosis care: in-patient estimated costs]." Rev Port Pneumol 9(2): 99-107.

[20] Greenberg, D., Y. Peterburg, et al. (2005). "Decisions to adopt new technologies at the hospital level: insights from Israeli medical centers." Int J Technol Assess Health Care 21(2): 219-227.

[21] Hazbon, M. H. (2004). "Recent advances in molecular methods for early diagnosis of tuberculosis and drug-resistant tuberculosis." Biomedica 24 Supp 1: 149-162.

[22] Hida, Y., K. Hisada, et al. (2012). "Rapid Diagnosis of Tuberculosis by using quenching probe PCR (GENECUBE(R))." J Clin Microbiol.

[23] Hughes, D. A., L. Tilson, et al. (2009). "Estimating drug costs in economic evaluations in Ireland and the UK: an analysis of practice and research recommendations." Pharmacoeconomics 27(8): 635-643.

[24] Jain, A., P. Dixit, et al. (2012). "Pre-XDR & XDR in MDR and Ofloxacin and Kanamycin resistance in non-MDR Mycobacterium tuberculosis isolates." Tuberculosis (Edinb) 92(5): 404-406.

[25] Kik, S. V., S. P. Olthof, et al. (2009). "Direct and indirect costs of tuberculosis among immigrant patients in the Netherlands." BMC Public Health 9: 283.

[26] King, S., S. Griffin, et al. (2006). "A systematic review and economic model of the effectiveness and cost-effectiveness of methylphenidate, dexamfetamine and atomoxetine for the treatment of attention deficit hyperactivity disorder in children and adolescents." Health Technol Assess 10(23): iii-iv, xiii-146.

[27] Kivihya-Ndugga, L. E., M. R. van Cleeff, et al. (2003). "A comprehensive comparison of Ziehl-Neelsen and fluorescence microscopy for the diagnosis of tuberculosis in a resource-poor urban setting." Int J Tuberc Lung Dis 7(12): 1163-1171.

[28] Kominski, G. F., S. F. Varon, et al. (2007). "Costs and cost-effectiveness of adolescent compliance with treatment for latent tuberculosis infection: results from a randomized trial." J Adolesc Health 40(1): 61-68.

[29] Kowada, A., G. A. Deshpande, et al. "Cost effectiveness of interferon-gamma release assay versus chest X-ray for tuberculosis screening of BCG-vaccinated elderly populations." Mol Diagn Ther 14(4): 229-236.

[30] Kowada, A., O. Takahashi, et al. (2008). "Cost effectiveness of interferon-gamma release assay for tuberculosis contact screening in Japan." Mol Diagn Ther 12(4): 235-251.

[31] Kritski, A. L., J. R. Lapa e Silva, et al. (1998). "Tuberculosis and HIV: renewed challenge." Mem Inst Oswaldo Cruz 93(3): 417-421.

[32] Lienhardt, C., P. Glaziou, et al. (2012). "Global tuberculosis control: lessons learnt and future prospects." Nat Rev Microbiol 10(6): 407-416.

[33] Lienhardt, C., M. Raviglione, et al. (2012). "New drugs for the treatment of tuberculosis: needs, challenges, promise, and prospects for the future." J Infect Dis 205 Suppl 2: S241-249.

[34] Mandalakas, A. M., A. C. Hesseling, et al. (2012). "Modelling the cost-effectiveness of strategies to prevent tuberculosis in child contacts in a high-burden setting." Thorax.

[35] Mason, A., H. Weatherly, et al. (2007). "A systematic review of the effectiveness and cost-effectiveness of different models of community-based respite care for frail older people and their carers." Health Technol Assess 11(15): 1-157, iii.

[36] Mehrotra, R., P. Metz, et al. (2002). "Comparison of in-house polymerase chain reaction method with the Roche Amplicor technique for detection of Mycobacterium tuberculosis in cytological specimens." Diagn Cytopathol 26(4): 262-265.

[37] Mitarai, S., A. Kurashima, et al. (2001). "Clinical evaluation of Amplicor Mycobacterium detection system for the diagnosis of pulmonary mycobacterial infection using sputum." Tuberculosis (Edinb) 81(5-6): 319-325.

[38] Nathanson, E., P. Nunn, et al. "MDR tuberculosis--critical steps for prevention and control." N Engl J Med 363(11): 1050-1058.

[39] Neves, L. A., S. R. Canini, et al. (2012). "[Aids and tuberculosis: coinfection from the perspective of the quality of life of patients]." Rev Esc Enferm USP 46(3): 704-710.

[40] Newhouse, J. P. (1992). "Medical care costs: how much welfare loss?" J Econ Perspect 6(3): 3-21.

[41] Pereira, S. M., M. L. Barreto, et al. (2012). "Effectiveness and cost-effectiveness of first BCG vaccination against tuberculosis in school-age children without previous tuberculin test (BCG-REVAC trial): a cluster-randomised trial." Lancet Infect Dis 12(4): 300-306.

[42] Perkins, M. D. (2000). "New diagnostic tools for tuberculosis." Int J Tuberc Lung Dis 4(12 Suppl 2): S182-188.

[43] Petitti, D. B. (2000). "Meta analysis, Decision Analysis, Cost-Effectiveness analysis. Methods for quantitative synthesis in medicine. ." New York Oxford University 2 ed.

[44] Polansky, F., O. Dymer, et al. (1968). "[Costs of tuberculosis control]." Cesk Zdrav 16(10): 543-549.

[45] Project, O. H. (2005). " Health Technologies and Decision Making. Organisation For Economic Co-Operation And Development. Paris, France."

[46] Ritchie, S. R., A. C. Harrison, et al. (2007). "New recommendations for duration of respiratory isolation based on time to detect Mycobacterium tuberculosis in liquid culture." Eur Respir J 30(3): 501-507.

[47] Rodrigues Vde, F., F. C. Queiroz Mello, et al. (2002). "Detection of Mycobacterium avium in blood samples of patients with AIDS by using PCR." J Clin Microbiol 40(6): 2297-2299.

[48] Roos, B. R., M. R. van Cleeff, et al. (1998). "Cost-effectiveness of the polymerase chain reaction versus smear examination for the diagnosis of tuberculosis in Kenya: a theoretical model." Int J Tuberc Lung Dis 2(3): 235-241.

[49] Rosen, V. M., D. C. Taylor, et al. (2010). "Cost effectiveness of intensive lipid-lowering treatment for patients with congestive heart failure and coronary heart disease in the US." Pharmacoeconomics 28(1): 47-60.

[50] Sanchez, J. I., L. Rossetti, et al. (2006). "Application of reverse transcriptase PCR-based T-RFLP to perform semi-quantitative analysis of metabolically active bacteria in dairy fermentations." J Microbiol Methods 65(2): 268-277.

[51] Sarmiento, O. L., K. A. Weigle, et al. (2003). "Assessment by meta-analysis of PCR for diagnosis of smear-negative pulmonary tuberculosis." J Clin Microbiol 41(7): 3233-3240.

[52] Scherer, L. C., R. D. Sperhacke, et al. (2011). "Comparison of two laboratory-developed PCR methods for the diagnosis of pulmonary tuberculosis in Brazilian patients with and without HIV infection." BMC Pulm Med 11: 15.

[53] Scherer, L. C., R. D. Sperhacke, et al. (2007). "PCR colorimetric dot-blot assay and clinical pretest probability for diagnosis of Pulmonary Tuberculosis in smear-negative patients." BMC Public Health 7: 356.

[54] Scherer, L. C., R. D. Sperhacke, et al. (2009). "Cost-effectiveness analysis of PCR for the rapid diagnosis of pulmonary tuberculosis." BMC Infect Dis 9: 216.

[55] Schijman, A. G., M. H. Losso, et al. (2004). "Prospective evaluation of in-house polymerase chain reaction for diagnosis of mycobacterial diseases in patients with HIV infection and lung infiltrates." Int J Tuberc Lung Dis 8(1): 106-113.

[56] Sharma, S. K., A. Mohan, et al. (2005). "Miliary tuberculosis: new insights into an old disease." Lancet Infect Dis 5(7): 415-430.

[57] Shi, L., M. Hodges, et al. (2010). "Good research practices for measuring drug costs in cost-effectiveness analyses: an international perspective: the ISPOR Drug Cost Task Force report--Part VI." Value Health 13(1): 28-33.

[58] Stafinski, T., D. Menon, et al. (2011). "To fund or not to fund: development of a decision-making framework for the coverage of new health technologies." Pharmacoeconomics 29(9): 771-780.

[59] Steffen, R., D. Menzies, et al. (2010). "Patients' costs and cost-effectiveness of tubercu-
      losis treatment in DOTS and non-DOTS facilities in Rio de Janeiro, Brazil." PLoS One
      5(11): e14014.

[60] Sul, S. o. H. P. o. S.-R. G. d. (2011). "Epidemilogical Report of Infective Diseases 2011."

[61] Taylor, R. S., M. F. Drummond, et al. (2004). "Inclusion of cost effectiveness in licens-
      ing requirements of new drugs: the fourth hurdle." BMJ 329(7472): 972-975.

[62] Tuberculose, I. C. B. d. (2004). "Diretrizes Brasileiras para Tuberculose." Jornal Brasi-
      leiro de Pneumologia 30(1).

[63] Udwadia, Z. F. (2012). "MDR, XDR, TDR tuberculosis: ominous progression." Thorax
      67(4): 286-288.

[64] van Cleeff, M., L. Kivihya-Ndugga, et al. (2005). "Cost-effectiveness of polymerase
      chain reaction versus Ziehl-Neelsen smear microscopy for diagnosis of tuberculosis
      in Kenya." Int J Tuberc Lung Dis 9(8): 877-883.

[65] Vassall, A., A. Seme, et al. (2010). "Patient costs of accessing collaborative tuberculo-
      sis and human immunodeficiency virus interventions in Ethiopia." Int J Tuberc Lung
      Dis 14(5): 604-610.

[66] Vassall, A., S. van Kampen, et al. (2011). "Rapid diagnosis of tuberculosis with the
      Xpert MTB/RIF assay in high burden countries: a cost-effectiveness analysis." PLoS
      Med 8(11): e1001120.

[67] Weatherly, H., M. Drummond, et al. (2009). "Methods for assessing the cost-effective-
      ness of public health interventions: key challenges and recommendations." Health
      Policy 93(2-3): 85-92.

[68] Weis, S. E., B. Foresman, et al. (1999). "Treatment costs of directly observed therapy
      and traditional therapy for Mycobacterium tuberculosis: a comparative analysis." Int
      J Tuberc Lung Dis 3(11): 976-984.

[69] WHO (2006). "Global tuberculosis control - surveillance, planning, financing" WHO
      Report 2006: 362.

Chapter 7

Pulmonary Tuberculosis in Latin America: Patchwork Studies Reveal Inequalities in Its Control – The Cases of Chiapas (Mexico), Chine (Ecuador) and Lima (Peru)

Héctor Javier Sánchez-Pérez, Olivia Horna–Campos,
Natalia Romero-Sandoval, Ezequiel Consiglio and
Miguel Martín Mateo

Additional information is available at the end of the chapter

1. Introduction

Tuberculosis (TB) has been present in Latin America since pre-historical times. Paleopathological studies have found signs of TB in mummies from many parts of the world. In fact, whenever human mummies have been found, signs of TB have been observed in bones, lungs or skin [1].

Although TB may be considered as nearly as old as humankind, the current epidemiological profile of this disease must not be considered as the natural or expected one, given the large numbers of prevalent and newly occurring cases. The main questions related with the persistence and rise of TB in many regions of Latin America, have to do with social processes and inequalities. In this sense, the different processes usually resulting in TB disease are directly related with social and economic behavior of human communities [1].

TB constitutes one of the most complex situations in the health field. This complexity both makes visible, and raises questions about the existing inequities in the political and socio-cultural structure and in class relations, as it is the result of the health-illness-care process. Among the main elements permitting operationalization of an analysis of this situation, we find social vulnerability and accessibility to a whole spectrum of health services (in geographical, cultural and economic terms), from opportunistic diagnosis to effective treatment (meaning cure).

In this sense, we understand as social vulnerability that set of economic, political, social and cultural conditions which determine that some individuals become infected by the TB bacillus while others do not, depending on the structural conditions which favor or hinder exposure to the disease,[1] as well as those differential aspects by which, among those infected, some get TB disease while others do not, and among those with TB disease some are cured (whether spontaneously or as a result of anti-TB treatment), others remain chronically ill (possibly with multi-drug resistance) while others die (generally those presenting the worst socioeconomic conditions and poorer health in general).

Nevertheless, TB prevention and control programmes are designed as if the disease behaved in a homogeneous way in all countries and regions, based almost solely on biological and medical factors, without taking into account socio-cultural, economic and political factors, such as poverty, malnutrition, health services accessibility and quality, as well as intra and inter-community political conflicts, among others.

This approach impedes acting on the particularities of marginal populations, which are precisely the ones presenting the highest rates of morbidity and mortality of this disease, manifesting various gradients of exposure and susceptibility. This leads governments to act on the basis of global estimates, even when their interpretation of these is limited and partial, because the differential exposures and true extent of TB are unknown.

Furthermore, this way of tackling TB does not reflect the reality of the different regions within a given country, because local or regional variations in rates of morbidity and mortality are disguised. Such variability could easily be quantified by, at the very least, providing the standard deviation corresponding to the global values of these rates for each country. Consequently, areas which should be given priority, paradoxically receive only limited resources for interventions.

In this sense, it is important to point out that TB, like HIV/AIDS, is one of the diseases for which estimations of impact in terms of incidence and prevalence are frequently based only on the registered cases. While it is true that published national and international figures often include estimates of sub-notification, they do not usually include gradients of the magnitude of the disease, or of the intra- or inter-regional under-notification rates, nor the differential rates between different population groups. According to several authors, calculation of the number of cases of TB disease is possible based on the expected evolution of cases of infection [2] or through linear regression modeling involving age-specific prevalence values across a range of differently aged populations [3]. Although this calculation technique for the frequency of TB and HIV status has been considered [4], there are currently no models in which population impact has been measured in terms of social factors.

In summary, in general terms, national and international policies to cope with TB ignore this reality, applying criteria of homogeneity in the calculation of objectives, materials, costs and logistics, among other aspects. While it is well known that marginal groups are the ones presenting the highest TB morbidity and mortality rates, their characterisation is not usually

---

1 According to World Health Organization calculations, one third to the human population is infected with TB bacillus

considered in the design of programmes for their prevention and control, so that TB continues to cause high rates of disease, death and ever-rising health costs in these groups, something which represents a violation of their human rights a consequence of governments having been incapable of preventing this situation.

Furthermore, the effectiveness of programs of TB Prevention and Control has been questioned because of their complexity. In this sense, a therapeutic intervention such as the Directly Observed Therapy – Short Course (DOTS) strategy, and socioeconomic and structural factors have been topics of discussion with regard the possible impact of one and the other, due to the decline of TB observed prior the use of antibiotics, as well as the goals met at present by DOTS strategy. In this regard, a correlation has been documented in Latin America between the early diagnosis of smear positive TB cases and improved cure rates [5]. So, one of the main emphasis of strategies to reduce the transmission of *Mycobacterium tuberculosis*, should be the identification of active TB cases, particularly in deprived and highly exposed populations.

The Africa and Latin America Research Groups Network (*Grups de Recerca d'America i Africa LLatines* -GRAAL) has conducted studies in marginal populations which reveal the conditions of patients, as well as the extent of the disease, of multi-drug resistance (MDR) and of mortality in these populations, producing figures which differ widely from the official average values. The main mechanism for tackling these aspects has been through doctoral theses. In this chapter we give examples of research undertaken in three different contexts of high poverty and social exclusion in Mexico, Ecuador and Peru.

2. Patch 1: Chiapas, Mexico

Chiapas is one of the poorest states in Mexico, and has one of the highest rates of indigenous margination as well as an acute lack of health care resources. According to official government statistics, Chiapas ranks almost last among all Mexican states in terms of health and socioeconomic indicators [6]. It is precisely in Chiapas where, due to the conditions of social exclusion, poverty, malnutrition and high mortality from infectious contagious diseases, the Zapatista National Liberation Army (EZLN) initiated an armed rising against the Mexican government in 1994, which drew attention, both nationally and internationally, to the precarious living and health conditions of the indigenous and peasant populations, not only in Chiapas, but throughout the entire country.

Several studies have been carried out by our team in areas of high levels of poverty in Chiapas: Our first attempt to analyze the pulmonary tuberculosis (PTB) situation arose out of the discovery that in the only hospital (Comitán General Hospital, Ministry of Health) in the region of the border with Guatemala for patients not covered by insurance (the majority of whom are indigenous),[2] there was empirical evidence of a high prevalence of PTB cases. In 1994, active case finding of patients with chronic cough (15 days or more) was carried out among all patients aged over 14 years seeking care in the hospital for whatever reason [7]. In this study

---

2 In Chiapas, over 80% of population is not covered by social security [6]

a rate of 21 positive PTB smears per hundred patients was found (95% CI=15.5-26.6), and the main factors associated with PTB were age (35-44 years), occupation (engaged in agricultural) and weight loss. Through a logistic regression model, we found that the subgroup of chronic cough patients aged 35-44 years, agricultural workers and who had lost weight, had the greatest likelihood of being PTB positive (68.7% compared to the overall average of 21% in the studied patients).

In addition, we noted that in the case of men, patients came to the hospital from near, far and very far distant communities, but in the case of women, the majority of them only came from communities which were near or very near. So we decided to carry out other studies in the hospital's area of influence, with the aim of analyzing factors related with the high PTB prevalence among users of secondary level care, not only in terms of health system aspects, but of demographic and socioeconomic characteristics:

a) In 1997 active case-finding was carried out among all patients aged over 14 years seeking consultation in a random sample of seven primary care centers [8]. We found a PTB positivity rate of 11.1 (95% CI=6.6-17.2) per hundred patients studied. The factors associated with PTB were size and poverty level of the locality of residence. Of the coughers identified, 56% sought care for non-respiratory symptoms.

b) In 1998 active case-finding was carried out among those aged over 14 years who had a cough of 15 days or more of duration, in a convenience sample of 1,894 households in 32 communities chosen at random based on the level of poverty and on travel time to reach the nearest health services (< 1 hour, 1 hour and over). In this study we found a rate of 276.9 per 100,000 persons studied (95%CI: 161-443) and that the only factor associated with PTB was blood in sputum, probably due to the homogenous conditions of extreme poverty among the populations studied [9].

Additionally, we found that the sensitivity of the smear testing was slightly lower than 50% in the primary care centers and in communities, and that the proportion of patients with active PTB that was receiving treatment was only 50% in the primary care centers, and 10.5% in the studied communities [10]. Also, we found high rates of anti-TB treatment defaulting [11], and very high levels of PTB multidrug-resistance (MDR): 4.6% and 29.2% primary and secondary MDR-TB, respectively. In fact, 14% of all studied PTB patients had MDR.

According to the logistic regression model fitted, the main variables associated with MDR were: having received anti-TB treatment previously, cough of three years or more of duration and not being indigenous. This is the only occasion in all our studies, which the condition of being indigenous appeared as a protective factor [12].

In 2000-2001 our team, together with Right to Health Defense Group and Physicians for Human Rights, carried out a population-based study to assess health conditions, and access to health services in the conflict zone initiated in 1994 between the EZLN and the Mexican government [6]. We found that the most affected regions by the armed conflict have fared even worse than the rest of Chiapas State. We performed a household survey in the municipalities most affected by the armed conflict among three types of communities: opposition communities, pro-government communities, and divided communities, i.e. which contained both opposition and pro-government groups.

This investigation identified serious deficiencies in both detection and treatment of PTB. In the 46 studied communities (n=2,997 households), we detected 29 cases of PTB among the population aged over 14 years. This means a rate of PTB of 85.3 per 100,000 in the general population, and of 161.2 among those aged 15 and older, almost three times the rate reported for the entire state. In this sense, only 13 (45%) cases of the 29 detected, had been identified by health services and were being treated. Of these 13 cases, one had not received any anti-TB treatment and six had defaulted from anti-TB treatment.

We also carried out two evaluations of a cohort of patients aged over 14 years diagnosed with PTB from January 1998 to July 2005, and found poor survival among them. In the first follow-up (performed during 2004-2006), the principal factors associated with PTB mortality were: age (45 years and over, OR=1.3; 95% CI=0.98-1.3), 0-3 years of schooling (OR=3.3; 95% CI=1.1-4.4), not living in the main village of their municipality (OR=1.2; 95% CI=1.0-1.3), living in a rural community (OR=2.7; 95% CI=1.1-6.8), not having been treated in DOTS (OR=1.2; 95% CI=1.0-1.3) and having defaulted from treatment (OR=11.5; 95% CI=5.3-24.8) [13].

In the second follow-up (carried out in 2008-2009), the factors associated with PTB mortality were age (45 years and over) and anti-TB treatment duration of under six months. The median survival time of those patients aged 45 and over who died was 718 days (range 0 to 3,185), while the median survival time in the reference group consisting of patients aged 15-34 years, was 688 days (range 8-1,841). With regard to the duration of anti-TB treatment, the median survival time among patients with incomplete treatment was 261 days (range 0-1,658), whereas among those dying in the reference group (with treatment completed), the median survival time was 1,137 days (range 202-3,185) [14].

The mortality rate in the patients studied was 4.6 per 100 person-years. Of the 78 deaths from PTB documented in this study, 25% occurred during the first six months following diagnosis (in other words, during treatment), 38% by the end of the first year from the date of diagnosis, 53% had died by the end of the second year, and 72% after three years.

The most important features of these studies are shown in Table 1.

3. Patch 2: Chine, Ecuador

During the decade from 1997 to 2006, inequalities of wealth and human development were extremely marked in Ecuador. The indigenous population, such as that residing in the central Andean province of Cotopaxi, has the highest poverty rates, and has many of its basic needs unmet. In Ecuador, up until 2006, the TB Prevention and Control Program was based on passive case finding of patients with respiratory symptoms (health personnel would check whether a patient visiting a health center had a productive cough of more than 15 days of duration). In contrast to what happens in cities, in rural areas the organization and functioning of the program relies on the presence of basic rural health teams; this means that is not uncommon for health personnel to be absent. This situation, among others, has resulted in TB notification being irregular. Although the average incidence reported is 65/100,000,[3] given the important level of under-reporting of TB cases, the true extent of the disease in Ecuador is unknown.

Setting	Frequency	Associated Factors
Chiapas, Mexico (only people 15 years of age and over)	Prevalence of PTB 21% in a hospital-based population with symptoms suggestive of TB	Association with age (35-44 years old), working in agricultural, and weight loss.
	Prevalence of PTB 11.1% among patients, consulting in primary health centers (PHC) with symptoms suggestive of TB	Association with poverty level
	Prevalence of PTB 277 per 100,000 persons studied in household surveys	Presence of blood in sputum; 50% of sensitivity in sputum test performed in PHC setting. High rate of defaulting treatment; and very high MDR-TB rates associated (by Logistic Regression) with previous PTB treatment, cough for more than 3 years and not being indigenous.
	Cohort of patients with PTB	Mortality was associated with poverty and deprivation characteristics and no access to DOTS.

Table 1. Pulmonary Tuberculosis (PTB) and associated factors observed within studies performed by GRAAL members in Mexico.

In Chine, an indigenous community of 653 inhabitants, in the parish of Angamarca, located in Cotopaxi Region, over 90% of its population have their basic needs unmet [15]. It is situated at an altitude of 3,500m above sea level and is two hours walk from the nearest health center, which during the period 2000 to 2004 was practically without staff. One of the co-authors of the present work (Natalia Romero) collaborated with the health team of this parish, during her period of rural medical training several years earlier. Following the diagnosis of one PTB case (the schoolmaster) in 2001, we conducted a study between 2001 and 2003, and found a prevalence rate of PTB-positive cases of 6.7% for the community as a whole [16].

On the basis of this single case, we saw the convenience of studying the total population of the community through a household survey (taking into account the experience obtained in Chiapas, México). The data collected was analyzed using the technique of multiple correspondence analyses, which allowed us to ascertain the risk and exposure factors in the community. All persons with chronic productive cough were asked to provide three sputum

3 World Health Organization. Ecuador: Health profile. Available at: http://www.who.int/countries/ecu/es/ (accessed 12 August 2012).

specimens. Given the degree of social and geographical exclusion of the community, PTB was diagnosed only by smear test.

Two hundred and two persons were identified with chronic cough (fifteen days or more), 173 of them, productive. Of 92 coughers in which it was possible analyze their sputum, 44 (48%) were PTB positive (representing 6.7% of the whole population and 11.3% of those aged 15 years and over). Among men, the highest prevalence was in the 35–44 age group (20.6%) and among women in the group aged ≥ 45 years (16.7%). Also, 27% of families had between one and four smear positive members. The factors associated with presence of PTB were: previous history of active TB (OR=6.0; 95% CI=2.9-12.3), haemoptysis (OR=3.8; 95% CI=1.5-10.0), and history of participating in seasonal migration (OR=2.44; 95% CI=0.91-6.54) [16].

With the intention of making some contribution to resolving the PTB problem, our team reached an agreement with the inhabitants of the community of Chine, in order to implement the DOTS strategy, while at the same time taking account of aspects of the community's world view. As consequence of this approach, we obtained a cure rate of 100%, confirmed by three negative smear-tests during the anti-TB treatment and cultures at the end of it (there were no defaults and no deaths) [17].

Although TB prevention and control programs encourage patients to visit health services and follow instructions, if they continue in their tendency to give little attention to socioeconomic, cultural and anthropological aspects, the results will be the same. How can better outcomes be expected if health services persist in acting as they always they do, including opening for restricted hours (from 8 am to 12 pm and from 2 to 6 pm)? In our intervention in Chine, symbolic referents, the religious dimension and rituals, as well as aspects of daily life (working hours, school, community and family calendar, seasonal migration, and traditional medical practices, among others) were taken into account.

The main results obtained in Ecuador, are shown in Table 2.

Chine, Cotopaxi, EcuadorPrevalence of PTB 6.7% in an entire indigenous community	PTB was associated with prior history of PTB (OR= 6.0; CI 95%: 2.9-12.3), with haemoptysis (OR= 3.8; CI 95%: 1.5-10.0).
	Cure rate of 100% based on community consent for the performing of DOTS strategy

CI: Confidence interval; OR: Odds Ratio

Table 2. Pulmonary Tuberculosis (PTB) and associated factors observed within studies performed by GRAAL members in Ecuador.

4. Patch 3: Lima, Peru

One of the coauthors of the present work (Olivia Horna), as a nurse responsible for coordinating the application of DOTS, realized that the TB Program was relaxing various aspects of the DOTS application, largely motivated by the economic conditions imposed in the area by the World Bank but also by recommendations from the Pan-American Health Organization itself: cessation of active case finding of coughers of 15 days or more on the grounds that the system was of low efficiency, and a switch to an ambulatory form of DOTS rather than in the patient's home, changes due to a shortage of funds to pay health technicians performing this function.

Given this situation combined with a feeling that the number of patients was rising at a higher rate than that calculated based on national rates, it was decided to perform a study to detect coughers of 15 days or more making use of the structure of the health system itself. The district of Ate-Vitarte was chosen to be targeted, since it consists mainly of lands occupied by migrants from the interior of the country, many forced off their lands due to violence between Peruvian armed forces and guerrilla movements from the interior, in particular Sendero Luminoso.

For this study, as in the cases of Chiapas, Mexico and of Chine, Ecuador, the health system approved and participated in order to guarantee anti-TB treatment and medical care for possible new cases identified by the study. Thus the same scheme was set up as employed previously in the outpatients department of Comitán hospital, whereby subjects recruited were people approaching the health system facilities in the area for medical care.

We interviewed 150 persons over 14 years of age who had productive chronic cough (fifteen days or more) seeking care in health services (primary care and hospitals). Of these, we obtained sputum samples from 142. The observed PTB prevalence rate was 12% [18], a figure very similar to that obtained in primary care centers in Chiapas (11%) [8]. None of the demographic or socioeconomic indicators analyzed were associated with PTB.

Of the variables studied, those found to be significantly associated with PTB, were: working away from home with respect those working at home (OR=6.99; 95% CI=0.89-54.61), persons commuting by minibuses compared with persons who used individual forms of transportation (OR=4.9; 95% CI=1.06-23.09), and commuting time one hour or more in a minibus (OR=3.35; 95% CI=1.12-10.1) [18].

Given the high prevalence of PTB in peripheral areas of Lima, as is the case of Ate-Vitarte District, and the results mentioned in the previous paragraph, we planned a study to determine whether the use of minibuses was associated with the spread of PTB. Commuting in these minibuses means that people travel in overcrowded situations with closed windows regardless of the weather, making trips of at least 30 minutes duration every day, in the company of TB patients going to a health center to receive DOTS treatment. Furthermore, if there is a strong association between using microbuses and the risk of infection, what would be expected among microbus drivers and fare-collectors that spend more than 8 hours per day in this environment?

Based on these precedents, we decided to carry out a study to assess infection by *Mycobacterium tuberculosis* and working conditions among workers of public transport [19]. In 2008 we performed a cross-sectional study with 104 workers from two public transport minibus companies of the Ate-Vitarte District. These minibus workers were interviewed and a tuberculin skin test (TST) administered. An induration greater than or equal to 10 mm was considered positive.

From these 104 workers, TST results were obtained for 73 (70.2%), of whom 56 (77%) were positive. We found that positivity was associated with the time they had worked on minibuses (more than two years, OR=11.04; 95% CI=3.17-38.43), and with working more than 60 hours per week (OR=9.8; 95% CI=2.85-33.72). This exposure gradient, a result of the working hours and time employed in the transport sector, stresses the importance of workers' job conditions.

Furthermore, strict revision of clinical histories of active TB patients in the health centers associated to the health districts of these workers, showed that standardized incidence rates for transport sector workers were 2.7- 4.5 times higher than those in the total working-age male and global populations of the health micro-network studied. The associations between TB and being a transport worker, and between MDR-TB and being a transport worker are both strong (OR 3.06, 95%CI 2.2-4.2 and OR 3.14, 95%CI 1.1-9.1, respectively). These results indicate that the use of informal public transport is a risk factor for TB infection and an occupational risk in countries with characteristics similar to those in Peru [20].

A summary of the main results obtained in Lima, is presented in table 3.

Lima, Peru	Incidence of PTB calculated within general population based on PHC micro-net data	TB associated with transport occupation (OR=3.06; CI 95%: 2.2-4.2) and with MDR-TB (OR= 3.14; CI 95%: 1.1-1.9)
	Prevalence of PTB 12% among commuters in a suburban area of Lima	Use of informal transport system: working away from home (OR= 6,99; CI 95%: 0.89-54.61; PPR = 6.06); commuting in minibuses (OR= 44.9; CI 95%: 1.06-23.09; PPR=4.09) and commuting more than one hour (OR=3.35; CI 95%: 1.12-10.1; PPR= 2.07)
	Prevalence of Mycobacterium Tuberculosis infection through PPD test of 77% among minibus drivers in informal transport	High work-related exposure: more than two years in job (OR= 11.04; CI 95%: 3.17-38.43) and working more than 60 hours per week (OR= 9.8; CI 95%: 2.85-33.72).

CI: Confidence interval; OR: Odds Ratio; PPR: Positive Prevalence Ratio

Table 3. Pulmonary Tuberculosis (PTB) and associated factors observed within studies performed by GRAAL members in Peru

5. The patchwork: What do these findings mean? Are they useful?

TB, far from being under control, as was believed at the end of the decade of the 1990s, continues to cause many deaths, disability, and health expenditure; indeed, it has been recognized that the situation may be worsening due to an accumulation of structural conditions favoring its appearance and development: increased poverty in important population nuclei (which are the most susceptible to the disease), migratory movements (whether due to economic, work, political or even environmental issues), higher incidence of other immuno-suppressive diseases (mainly HIV/AIDS and diabetes), or weakening of health of certain individuals (such as due to malnutrition, and chronic pneumopathies), the increasingly more common appearance of forms of MDR, and the shortage of health resources to cope with TB, mainly in areas of greater socioeconomic exclusion. In this sense, the so-called developed countries have also felt the impacts of the disease, largely due the appearance of HIV/AIDS and to cases among immigrants who, whether legally or illegally, settle in foreign territories seeking to improve on the conditions which caused them to leave their places of origin.[4] These populations are generally speaking the most socioeconomically disadvantaged groups.

There is no doubt that TB is an outcome indicator of the socioeconomic, cultural and political structure of a population. TB is a historical reflection of the forms of social construction, particularly of the post-industrial revolution era experienced in capitalist countries. TB in this sense feeds, to a greater or lesser degree, depending on circumstances, on the social context in order to reproduce, and this fact finds expression, as documented in the present studies, in various gradients of exposure and susceptibility to the disease, in which the more socioeco-nomically disadvantaged groups are the ones most affected by the disease, but the ones which, paradoxically, usually receive least attention, whether in terms of prevention, diagnosis, or treatment, and hence cure rates are low.

Two million people die every year from TB, the majority of them in the "under-developed countries". The Global Plan to Stop TB 2006-2015 aims to treat 50 million people, save 14 million lives, and expand equitable access to quality diagnosis and treatment. According to this Global Plan, by 2010 it was expected "to be using diagnostic test that allow rapid, sensitive and inexpensive detection of active TB… and introduce the first new TB drug in 40 years. It also expects to see a new, safe, effective and affordable vaccine available by 2015" [21]. However, the World Health Organization, Pan-American Health Organization and Governments in general, establishing targets for TB control programs, take as their basis the reports they receive from the countries themselves, with the result that programs elaborated are eminently political, whose objectives and information basis constitute a kind of feedback system which rapidly departs from reality.

TB control programs thus planned are designed as though the social structure of the countries was homogeneous, and this impedes acting in such a way as to take account of the particu-larities of marginal populations, which are the ones presenting the highest rates of prevalence of this disease. The usual ways of working lead to government planning and actions being based on central estimates and tackling of global objectives. For example, the global medium-term goal for TB control is to halve TB prevalence and death rates by 2015 as compared to 1990 levels, and to achieve a reduction in its incidence, as part of the Millennium Development Goals (number six) [22,23].

---

4 The first report of a rise in cases of HIV/AIDS was published in 1991, affecting New York City, and the status of TB was changed to that of an AIDS-defining disease, although it has been calculated that currently 50% of new TB cases in the European Union occur among immigrants.

This type of planning and programming of objectives apparently does not take account of the particular situations affecting the population, above all those aspects which are notably different from the global mean values. In fact the few population based studies available, some involving Latin American countries, likewise fail to treat marginal populations specially. For example, if it was not for international support, few governments would have sufficient resources to conduct national health surveys, which are usually carried out through household interviews, based on self-perceived morbidity, and which hardly ever include laboratory tests to identify diseased individuals (TB in our case). Generally, the level of disaggregation of surveys of this type goes no further than large geographical regions (north, south, east, etc), tending to disguise inter- and intra-regional heterogeneity, and the data are analyzed based on artificially created convenience categories, not based on observed patterns of disease or deaths.

In other words, it is usual that global policies emanating from the international agencies and institutions ignore the true situation, applying criteria of homogeneity in the calculation of targets, costs of equipment and supplies and staffing levels, among other aspects. Curiously, despite it being well known that social factors are related with TB, they are not taken into consideration in order to improve the quality of plans to control it.

In order to identify, analyze and ideally contribute alternative solutions to the problem of unmet needs of socioeconomically excluded populations, means working with samples which are not representative of the general population, but rather focused on these sub-populations, biased precisely due to their conditions. In this sense, our team has been employing the patchwork approach, involving studies focusing on marginal or susceptible populations, those with the worst socioeconomic and health conditions. In the case of TB, these circumstances (poverty, social vulnerability, and shortage of health facilities) are well recognized as one of the basic determinants of the presence and spread of the disease, but its characterization usually is not considered by health systems in their solution proposals [24].

For example, in marginalized rural areas, in the best case, active TB case finding is limited in practice, to identifying chronic coughers among users who seek health care. This results in at least three possible situations: a) there may be delays in the TB diagnosis (patients arrive in an advanced stage of the disease);[5] if the medical consultation is for reasons other than respiratory symptoms, TB may not even be detected;[6] and, c) that a certain proportion of patients do not use the health services (due to accessibility barriers which may be geographical, economic or cultural)[7] and hence are not even diagnosed [10].

---

5 Several studies have shown that groups living in conditions of greater socioeconomic margination present longer delays in seeking care for health problems [26,27].

6 In several studies we found that PTB status is not associated with the reason for visiting health services [10].

7 Political conflicts (belonging to a particular organization), religious conflicts (not belonging to the religion predominant in the community), administrative barriers (nearest clinic not the one assigned officially), and conflicts deriving from access to and utilization of natural resources (water, timber, etcetera) can mean that certain individuals are denied access to health services, or they are denied medical care or drugs [6].

In this context, women living in remote and marginalized regions, have a more pronounced lack of access to health services due to gender reasons: there are differences in the process of seeking medical care, and in the quality of the care received between women and men [25].

Furthermore, in Chiapas, Ecuador and Peru, as in many other regions of Latin America, TB cases notified to the information systems of the health sector, and from which incidence rates are estimated, correspond to cases detected in health services by acid-fast bacilli. We have documented that in rural and marginalized areas, its sensitivity is around 50%. This is an important aspect to consider because health system detection of TB cases is based on smear testing, meaning that in marginalized communities many cases are not detected. In consequence, the target of detecting at least 75% of cases is far from being reached, implying the presence of a not unappreciable risk of transmission of TB [9]. Indeed, the detection rate in hospitals studied in Chiapas is below this figure of 75%. The suboptimal case detection rate reflects an inadequate of quality medical care, probably health personnel are often overwhelmed by daily activities, as well as insufficiently trained, motivated, aware, and remunerated [10].

In order to increase detection rates, as it was demonstrated, the health system must take into account the considerable difficulties involved in obtaining and analyzing sputum samples in marginalized areas: cultural barriers (language spoken, world view) and economic barriers, as well as technical problems to be overcome in order to obtain adequate quantity and quality of sputum samples. It is therefore necessary to reduce the cultural and socioeconomic barriers between health care providers and people [10]. Not surprisingly, some results of our investigations show that apart from cultural barriers, there are also structural barriers [11].

In the same way, we have found that a very low proportion of patients eligible for anti-TB treatment effectively receive such treatment, and very high proportions of treatment failures and incomplete follow-up [10].

Two further aspects deserve special attention in the context of the studies conducted in Chiapas, Mexico, as well as in Peru: the problem of MDR, and the high mortality among patients diagnosed of PTB. Both indicators constitute expressions of the complete failure of the health system which, for whatever reason, did not manage to adequately treat these people, who consequently either died of TB, or were left as chronic MDR cases (which would lead to their death also, sooner or later).

In the case of MDR, it is well documented that the vast majority of cases of this type result from inappropriate treatment and follow up by the health system. According to official statistics, worldwide, the rates of MDR recorded in 2009 and 2010 were the highest ever, and trends in MDR rates are unclear in the majority of countries [28]. The observed rates of MDR in Chiapas suggest that in marginalized and excluded regions, it is a serious public health problem of alarming proportions. While the MDR rates calculated for the country as a whole are 1-3% for primary, and 20% for secondary MDR, in our studies these rates were 4.6% and 29%, respectively [12].

Although our results were made known to the health authorities, there are no signs to suggest that the TB situation has improved: the health system continues failing to diagnose cases appropriately and application of the DOTS strategy is very deficient: even if TB patients are diagnosed, in many cases they begin, but do not complete their anti-TB treatment. In this sense, we must emphasize the following aspects:

a. It is extremely difficult to perform culture analysis, in order to determine MDR status, in a patient with less than six months of treatment, due to poor quality sputum samples. The main obstacles to obtaining good quality sputum samples are: barriers in communication with indigenous people, distance of the communities from the centers where samples are processed, unsuitable transport conditions of samples (risk of exposure to sunlight or lack refrigeration), among others.

b. It is very plausible that in indigenous populations, due to their having less contact with health services, there are more undiagnosed TB cases and that, among non-indigenous patients, more TB cases are diagnosed but not necessarily treated adequately [12].

c. A patient confirmed with MDR condition, is practically impossible to treat, given the high cost of the secondary treatment, and because if the health system is incapable of guaranteeing the follow up of a patient sensitive to the four primary drugs during six months, it is probably even less able to follow up a MDR patient not only in terms of the time required (from 6 months to 1.5 or 2 years) but also in terms of level of patient care, due to the possible secondary effects of the "second line drugs" employed. In this sense, if a program cannot guarantee appropriate follow up and compliance with treatment among TB patients, it should not initiate their treatment, thus condemning them to a situation of no hope of cure, with all that this implies, not only for the patient, but also for his family, who apart from watching their family member suffer, are also exposed to the possibility of their catching the disease.

With regard to mortality due to TB, we have found unacceptably high rates. In addition, a considerable proportion of TB patients die without having received any medical care.[8] We found that 55% of patients whose death was related to TB, had died within two years of being diagnosed, possibly due to delays in diagnosis, and the poor quality of the follow-up in their anti-TB treatment. Whereas the life expectancy in Chiapas is 72.2 years [29], the average age of deceased patients was 47.4 years, representing an average of at least 24 potential years of life lost [13]. We believe that the accumulation of unfavorable living conditions such as malnutrition, poverty, as well as deficient and/or lack of health services, makes them an especially vulnerable group. According to official statistics, while in 2009 the PTB mortality for the country was 1.7/100,000 inhabitants in Chiapas it was 3.79 with the same denominator [14].

Our findings have provided evidence that in the area studied, patients being aged 45 years and over, not having completed the established six months of treatment, and not having been treated via the DOTS strategy, are all associated with a higher risk of the patient dying from PTB.

---

8 Eighteen percent of patients traced to their homes, in a study carried out in Chiapas, had died. Of the 40 deaths presumed to have been associated with PTB, 33 died without having received medical care [13]

Based on our findings, we can say that people from rural and indigenous communities suffer mistreatment by the health services [30], meaning, among other aspects, deficient application of the DOTS strategy (sometimes due to shortages in the supply of anti-TB drugs [31], or poor follow up), leading to higher mortality and increasing their chances of becoming MDR cases [12,13].

Another fact that reduces the chances of successfully carrying out patient follow up, is migratory movements. Migration in the region is mainly due to economic factors, but can also be for health reasons. Sometimes patients are registered by health services as urban patients when in fact they are not, or they give a false address in order to obtain the first consultation, but subsequently return to their rural communities or find another place to live without notifying the health services.

In addition, health services give little consideration to socio-cultural and anthropological aspects. For example, in indigenous medicine the process of health and illness involves their world view, their personal and community histories, in an atmosphere of trust in which supernatural intervention, transgression of social norms, culpability, or malice on the part of enemies, are all admissible possible causes of the disease [16,32,33]. In this sense, patients may seek care from traditional medicine practitioners, who attend them in accordance with their age-old diagnostic and therapeutic rituals.

On the other hand, the use of public transport is a risk factor of TB not only among users, but also among minibus drivers and fare-collectors, and hence may be considered an occupational disease in these workers, who work in conditions such that not only do they have precarious employment, with all its implications (temporary contract, no social security or medical insurance, among other aspects) but also their job places them in a position of greater vulnerability to TB, since if they don't work, they don't get paid, and hence it is very probable that many of them go to work despite their illness, if they are able to do so, only seeking care when the disease really makes it impossible for them to continue working. In this sense, a worker with active PTB is a source of infection not only for co-workers but also for passengers. In countries where TB is endemic with increased circulation of resistant mycobacteria, the situation could be even worse. In a situation of this kind, the health system should be implementing, at very least, home-based DOTS to avoid exposure as far as possible, as well as implementing specifically designed occupational health programs [19,20,34].[9]

Observation of the particular facts which determine the appearance of TB and its prognosis, shows that the diagnosis and treatment strategies employed by the health services are just that, strategies, rather than ends in themselves, something which, unfortunately, is frequently emphasized. If more clearly focused measures are not taken, TB will not disappear in marginalized areas, despite the fact that trends in the ecological indices suggest that TB is tending to decline in Latin American countries; rather, it will persist as a greater public health problem for years to come.

---

9 In fact, the authors believe that more attention ought to be given to the risk of infection, by any aerially transmitted disease that utilization of public transport represents, for both passengers and the workers.

Pulmonary Tuberculosis in Latin America: Patchwork Studies Reveal Inequalities
in Its Control – The Cases of Chiapas (Mexico), Chine (Ecuador) and Lima (Peru)

191

In our view, to remain with the idea that TB is decreasing in Latin America, tends to conceal the failure which the rise in MDR patients represents. In any case, countries are alarmed by the rise in MDR because of the cost of treatment and its inefficiency, not necessarily for the health and welfare of TB patients, particularly if they are poor, as our studies suggest.

One discussion point is clear. Objective-oriented programs which attribute to the entire country the same values of incidence and detection rates present a problem known as "trimmed estimation", meaning that when the established objectives are reached, case finding and detection are relaxed, or the resources to permit continuing with case finding and/or provision of treatment, are cut short.

If, together with these data we take into account cases in areas enjoying lower TB incidence, and if this total was the true number of existing cases, the result would necessarily be a systematic reduction in incidence rates, leading to false optimism, whose historical cost has been a relaxation of efforts to prevent and control TB worldwide during the decade of the 1980s of last century.

Imagine the simple case that we have an incidence rate of X, in a given country. This figure conditions the work plan for the coming year in terms of supplies, staff, anti-TB treatment drugs, etcetera. Later on, 70% of the reporting areas indicate a rate of 0.9X, another 15% of areas a rate of X, and the remaining 15% provide no data on rates, but their population is taken into account in the denominator. The final rate for this country, based on these hypothetical figures, would be 0.78X. In other words, not receiving reports from the areas with the worst conditions provokes an apparent reduction in the global rate.

Unfortunately, even without questioning the figures declared, we know that areas which do not report (or report, but at best with high levels of under-notification) are the ones with the poorest conditions, both in terms of the socioeconomic conditions of the population which theoretically must be cared for, and in terms of the lack of resources and other failures in the organization and functioning of the program. Thus, by apparently having fewer cases, the resources dedicated to the TB prevention and control program are also cut back, and this creates a vicious circle which is difficult to break, so that program outcomes may be false, i.e. underestimates of the numbers of cases.

There is therefore a clear need to promote studies specifically aiming to analyze the population groups most vulnerable to TB, and in this way ascertain more precisely their situation, even when they are not representative of what happens in a given country. Continuing to carry out representative population based studies can only yield the probably already known rate for the country as a whole, and the situation of marginal groups will not be reflected in such rate.

In this sense, the patchwork studies contribute very valuable elements which help to make more visible and understandable the situation of population groups which go unnoticed in the global rates utilized in public health. We would encourage potentiating studies which break with the classical schemes, and use methods appropriate for the analysis of samples considered too small by classical approaches, but without renouncing the maximum of scientific rigor, as demonstrated by the doctoral theses developed in projects conducted in the three settings we have dealt with, Chiapas (Mexico), Chine (Cotopaxi,

Ecuador), and Lima (Peru), and whose results have been published in journals of medium and high impact factor.

On the other hand, Ecuador and Peru present changes in their control program strategies: active case finding, incorporation of economic incentives, strategies to reduce stigma among patients, citizens' observatories and integration of TB research in academic circles, among other aspects. It will be fundamental to perform studies which evaluate possible effects of such changes.

As the studies have shown, a failure to introduce changes in the structure and functioning of TB prevention and control programs would have as a consequence that this disease will continue to severely affect the most marginalized sectors of society:

In the field of TB prevention, several authors recognize that effective efforts have not yet been fully considered, and that it is necessary to improve this issue, for example through better vaccines and better chemotherapy for preventive treatment [22].

In the field of TB diagnosis, efforts must be made to reinforce active case finding of coughers, as for example, incorporating other diagnostic tests which allow better detection of the disease (from the use of cultures, and conducting molecular tests, to the search for faster diagnostic methods, such as biosensors). Epidemiological surveillance systems rely on smear testing, failing to take into account that in marginalized and rural areas these tests with only around 50% sensitivity, leave large numbers of cases undetected by the health services, or who will only be captured in advanced stages of the disease [12-14]. It is not unusual to find, within a given Latin American country, that while highly developed regions have advanced technologies available for TB diagnosis, in others the only possibility for diagnosis is the smear test. Nor is it unusual in regions of this type to find that smear testing is done badly, both in numerical terms (hardly ever obtaining three samples from a given patient), and in terms of quality (for reasons attributable to the poor quality of samples, such as errors in collection, storage, transport, processing and reading of results) [10,35].

In regard to anti-TB treatment, while the DOTS strategy has achieved a certain level of effectiveness in curing patients and saving lives, the epidemiological impact has so far been less than predicted [22], perhaps among other reasons, because treatment programs do not find patients soon enough to significantly reduce transmission [5]. Thus it is necessary to ensure: a) training, awareness and supervision of health personnel about the importance of avoiding patients defaulting from treatment, as well as guaranteeing the appropriate supply of medication; b) when necessary to adapt the DOTS strategy, both socially and culturally, taking into account the community health agents, community world view, and implementing the scheme in the patient's homes, supporting them and their families economically during their treatment; and c) that patients and their family are accompanied during the six months of treatment, in order to cope with possible secondary effects and to overcome possible barriers (alcoholism, religion, gender issues, seasonal migration, etcetera) which make compliance with anti-TB treatment difficult.

6. Conclusions: Tuberculosis as indicator of structural violence and violations of human rights

One of the main aspects we want to stress in the present work is the fact that analyzing TB through the measurement of global indicators conceals the situation of vulnerability to the disease suffered by socioeconomically disadvantaged population groups. The data obtained in the different studies we have presented show that there is a need for methodological approaches (such as that known as patchwork studies) which allow the measurement and analysis of the distribution of TB among different population groups.

It is well known that TB is one of the infectious diseases which has caused the most deaths among humans [36], above all among the socioeconomically most vulnerable groups [37]. These groups, apart from having higher risks of infection, developing active disease, and dying due to TB, are also the ones facing the greatest barriers (including information barriers) to access health services [38]. In this sense, and given that nowadays the medical resources to cure the disease are available, the fact that even today TB continues to cause deaths may be considered as an indicator of the violation of human rights in excluded and marginalized populations, as well as an indicator of "structural violence", given that it is precisely the social, economic, cultural and political structures which do not allow certain social groups to achieve their full potential, while other groups do so, due to the unequal distribution of power and available resources, placing some in conditions of social privilege and others in situations of social vulnerability [39].

The social context of TB is strongly related with social justice. The history of TB teaches us that the improvement of social conditions, work conditions ant the access to better quality food decreased its mortality in the pre-microbial stage [40].

Taking as a starting point that the appearance, development and distribution of TB is largely influenced by social determinants, and that public health achievements will depend on actions outside the health care sector [41], two forms of interventions are necessary: a) those reducing peoples' vulnerability, such as poor living and working conditions, and improving nutrition, among other aspects (such as structural and socioeconomic conditions), and b) by seeking alternatives that promote higher levels of prevention, diagnosis and cure of TB.

Two clear examples that help to visualize health related inequalities in respect to TB are firstly, the so-called "10/90 gap", in reference to the fact that only 10% of worldwide expenditure on health research and development is devoted to the problems primarily affect the poorest 90% of the world's population, and that 90% of worldwide expenditure is devoted to the problems that affect the richest 10% of the world's population.

The second example is the comparison between HIV-AIDS and TB. Whereas the first cases of HIV-AIDS were described during the decade of the 1980s of the last century, today it is one of the diseases which have received the most resources for its prevention and treatment, and notable advances have been achieved in these aspects, and in improving survival of patients. At the end of the last century, it was practically a death sentence, and yet today we have a series of drugs which increase both survival and quality of life of these patients.

In contrast, despite the fact that TB has been accompanying humans for thousands of years, and that the etiological agent was first described in 1882, it is the disease which has alone caused the greatest numbers of deaths in the adult population worldwide, and for which the resources currently dedicated are insufficient to lead us to expect, in the foreseeable short or medium term, the appearance of more effective measures for its control. Perhaps this is because it is considered a disease of the poor, and thus there is no incentive to "invest" in it? As some of our colleagues have pointed out: "even if the Global Plan to Stop TB is successfully implemented and results in the expected rate of reduction in incidence of about 6%, the global incidence rate in 2050 would still be of the order of 100 per million of inhabitants, i.e. about 100 times greater than the elimination target" [22].

From the viewpoint of international human rights law, by providing woefully substandard health services to marginalized populations, and failing to assure prevention of disease through appropriate public health measures, governments violate their obligations in human rights [6].

In this sense, high rates of TB constitute a reflection of the fact that certain populations face important obstacles in their exercise of the right to health, and other economic, social and cultural rights, due to the main social determinants of this disease being associated to social exclusion and poverty [31]. The presence of TB constitutes a violation of the right to the highest attainable standard of physical and mental health ("the right to health protection") which is inextricably related to the right to life and other human rights that allow an individual to live with dignity [6,42].

The International Covenant on Economic, Social and Cultural Rights (ICESCR) in its Article 12, Paragraph 2, sets out the steps states should take in order to fulfill the highest attainable standard of health, and includes "the prevention, treatment and control of epidemic, endemic, occupational and other diseases, as well as the creation of conditions which would assure to all medical service and medical attention in the event of sickness".

The General Comment issued by the Economic, Social and Cultural Rights Committee [43], establishes that "the underlying determinants of health, such as including adequate sanitation facilities, hospitals, clinics and other health related buildings, trained medical and professional personnel" have to be available in sufficient quantity with the States parties, and specifies that health facilities, goods and services must be available, accessible, acceptable and of adequate quality.

In this General Comment, accessibility has four overlapping dimensions [43, paragraph 12 (b)]:

First, the principle of non-discrimination,[10] on the grounds of sex (poorer quality of care among women than men), ethnic group (patients from indigenous communities receive poorer care), color, political filiation (belonging or not to the dominant political party in a region can affect access to care and to medication), religion (care may be denied to community members not belonging to the dominant religion), physical or mental disability, health status, sexual

---

10 Non-discrimination is a core principle for the full realization of the right to health, as for all human rights [6]

orientation, among others. A violation occurs when there is the intention or effect of nullifying or impairing the equal enjoyment or exercise of the right to health [43, paragraph 18].

Second, physical accessibility, meaning that health facilities, goods and services must be within safe physical reach for all groups, specially the vulnerable or marginalized ones, such as ethnic and indigenous populations.

Third, economic accessibility requires that health facilities, goods and services must be affordable for all, including socially disadvantaged groups. It points out that poorer persons should not be disproportionately burdened with health expenses, and those individuals (e.g. peasants) who through not having access to cash face particular difficulties, need to be considered in governmental policy and practice.

Fourth, the right to seek, receive and impart information and ideas concerning health issues, which includes health information in indigenous languages.

With regard to acceptability, it is understood that "health facilities, goods and services must be respectful of medical ethics and culturally appropriate… [and] requires respect for traditional medicines and practices which have not been shown to be harmful to human health" [43, paragraph 12 (c)].

For adequate quality, it requires that health facilities, goods and services must be scientifically and medically appropriate and of good quality (skilled medical personnel, scientifically approved and unexpired drugs, and hospital equipment, among other aspects) [43, paragraph 12 (d)].

Unfortunately, the findings of our studies indicate that health care is not sufficiently available or accessible (in either quantity or quality) to more disadvantaged social groups, creating mistrust among them of the government health services, something that is reflected in the relatively high percentage of people that do not use these services, even for vaccinations. This situation is more marked when health services are not culturally adapted, when people perceive mistreatment on the basis of their ethnicity or social conditions and health personnel make disparaging remarks about their habits and demeanor [6].

Other indicators of violation of human rights in TB patients are:

- Failure to improve the level of health in a population. The fact that health indicators, in our case indicators of TB do not improve in a population, even though they do not worsen, constitutes a violation of human rights (specifically of the right to "Non-retrogression and Adequate Progress").

- The presence of inequalities in access to quality and coverage of health services (in the case of TB affecting aspects from prevention to cure).

- The lack of meaningful popular participation, in regard to the making of decisions which involve the design, organization and functioning of health services. It is common to find that local health services nominate a "health promoter", charged with various activities such as vaccination, routine pediatric checkups, etcetera, but this does not necessarily mean the community has a voice or participates in the definition of its own priorities, decision-making in regard to planning of activities or elaboration and evaluation of health programs for the community. Veneklasen and colleagues have said [44]: "True rights-based participation requires programs that enable people to be active, informed and critical agents and citizens, rather than objects of charity". In this sense, the International Labor Organization, Convention 169 [45] stresses that health services shall, to the extent possible be, "planned and administered in co-operation with the peoples concerned and take into account their economic, geographical, social and cultural conditions as well as their traditional preventive care healing practices and medicines".

- The lack of accountability in health programs, which in addition are usually not evaluated. In this sense, the fact that a person is not treated appropriately by the health services, which in itself constitutes a violation of his right to health, should also imply a right to compensation by the State, which could take the form of restoration of his health, economic compensation, satisfaction or guarantees that the situation will not be repeated. On the other hand, if it is true that more resources are needed, they must be spent in such a way as to foster self-sufficiency and reduce inequities. Greater health care expenditure does not necessarily reduce inequalities [5].

- This dimension is also related to the enactment and enforcement of laws to provide sanctions for gender based violence or sexual abuse of women patients by health personnel, as well as people affected by mistrust. In addition, a legal framework must be adopted to operationalize the protection of patient human rights in the health services, establishing mechanisms for monitoring their compliance. The figure of a human rights ombudsman is a good example for monitoring, to investigate and sanction perpetrators in cases of abuse or malpractice and medical negligence claims [6].

- The lack of multi-sectorial strategies. Governmental programs should not compete among themselves, but rather be designed inter alia to promote health services, improve adequate dwelling conditions, education, work, and adequate nutrition. Until this happens, the plight of marginalized populations will persist. In the last instance, violations of the Economic, Social and Cultural Rights occur "when a state fails to satisfy a minimum core obligation to ensure the satisfaction of, at very least, minimum essential levels of the rights" [46].

- The lack of access to health information. Social participation and monitoring are impossible without access to information. This implies that governments should collect data on a disaggregated basis (by ethnicity, gender, socio-economic status, language, among other aspects) and this information, together with the methodologies used, must be readily available to the public. Of course, it also includes the right of TB patients to see their medical records, to give informed consent in all procedures, and to confidential management of their disease.

The performance of patchwork studies has allowed us to identify, evaluate and measure the situation of marginalized population groups in three different contexts (Chiapas, Mexico; Chine, Cotopaxi, Ecuador and Lima, Peru). Our findings revealed the poor quality of diagnosis and treatment of TB patients. Our data can be useful not only in the studied regions, but also in other countries with similar socioeconomic inequalities, if they are taken into account by the health authorities in order to provide all people (especially the more socially vulnerable groups) with: effective prevention programs, a reliable and timely diagnosis, adequate anti-TB treatment and follow-up, clear and appropriate information and counseling about TB (what it is, mechanisms of transmission and possibility of infecting others, etcetera).

In consequence it is necessary change the dysfunctional health system that contributes to the persistence and intensification of exclusion, voicelessness, and inequity, while simultaneously defaulting on its potential and obligation to fulfill human rights and contribute to the building of more equitable, egalitarian and democratic societies. The history of TB teaches us that the improvement of social justice led to increase the global health conditions and thus, it avoids the called "social diseases", including TB. The academic community has much to say and actively contribute in these aspects. The first step is to do research in order to make visible excluded people. To analyze, sensitize and lead to better socioeconomic conditions is an assignment for all of us.

Author details

Héctor Javier Sánchez-Pérez[1], Olivia Horna–Campos[2,3], Natalia Romero-Sandoval[4], Ezequiel Consiglio[1,5] and Miguel Martín Mateo[2]

*Address all correspondence to: hsanchez@ecosur.mx

*Address all correspondence to: ohornac@yahoo.es

*Address all correspondence to: natalia.romero.15@gmail.com

*Address all correspondence to: econsiglio_ar@hotmail.com

*Address all correspondence to: miquel.martin@uab.es

1 Society, Culture and Health Academic Area, The College of the Southern Border (ECO-SUR), San Cristóbal de Las Casas, Chiapas, The Africa and Latin America Research Groups Network (GRAAL)-ECOSUR, Mexico

2 The Africa and Latin America Research Groups Network (GRAAL). Faculty of Medicine, Biostatistics Unit, Barcelona Autonomous University, Bellaterra, Spain

3 Barcelona Public Health Agency, Epidemiology Service, Barcelona, Spain

4 School of Medicine, Pontificia Universidad Católica del Ecuador, Quito, The Africa and Latin America Research Groups Network - GRAAL-ECUADOR, Ecuador

5 University Institute of Health, National University of La Matanza, San Justo, Buenos Aires, Argentina

References

[1] Gómez i Prat J & Mendoza de Souza SMF (2003). Prehistoric Tuberculosis in America: Adding Comments to a Literature Review. Mem Inst Oswaldo Cruz, Rio de Janeiro, Brasil 2003; 98(Suppl. I): 151-159.

[2] Baez-Saldana R, Perez-Padilla JR, Salazar Lezama MA. Discrepancias entre los datos ofrecidos por la Secretaría de Salud y la Organización Mundial de la Salud sobre tuberculosis en México, 1981-1998. Salud Pública Mex 2003; 45: 78-83.

[3] Barroto Gutiérrez S, Armas Perez L, González Ochoa, Peláez Sánchez O, Arteaga Yero AL, Sevy Court J. Distribución y tendencia de la tuberculosis por grupos de edades y por municipios en Ciudad de La Habana, Cuba (1986-1998). Rev Espe Salud Pública 2000; 74: 507-515.

[4] Dolin PJ, Raviglione MC, Kochi A. Global tuberculosis incidence and mortality during 1990-2000. Bull World Health Org 1994; 72: 213-220.

[5] Dye C, Lönnroth K, Jaramillo E, Williams BG, Raviglione M. Trends in tuberculosis incidence and their determinants in 134 countries. Bull World Health Organ 2009; 87: 683-691.

[6] Sánchez-Pérez HJ, Arana-Cedeño M, Yamín AE. Excluded people, eroded communities. Realizing the right to health in Chiapas, Mexico. Phycisians for Human Rights, Boston, Massachussets: El Colegio de la Frontera Sur, Centro de Capacitación en Ecología y Salud para Campesinos – Defensoría del Derecho a la Salud; 2006.

[7] Sánchez-Pérez HJ, García GM, Halperin D. Pulmonary tuberculosis in the border region of Chiapas, Mexico. Int J Tuberc Lung Dis 1998;2(1):37-43.

[8] Sánchez-Pérez HJ, Prat-Monterde D, Jansá JM, Martín-Mateo M. Tuberculosis pulmonar y uso de servicios del primer nivel de atención en zonas de alta y muy alta marginación socioeconómica de Chiapas, México. Gaceta Sanitaria (España) 2000;14(4):268-276.

[9] Sánchez-Pérez HJ, Flores-Hernández JA, Jansá JM, Caylá JA, Martín-Mateo M. Pulmonary tuberculosis and associated factors in areas of high levels of poverty in Chiapas, Mexico. International Journal of Epidemiology. 2001;30:386-393.

[10] Sánchez-Pérez HJ, Hernán M, Hernández-Díaz S, Jansá JM, Halperin D, Ascherio A. Detection of pulmonary tuberculosis in Chiapas, Mexico. Annals of Epidemiology 2002; (12)3:166-172.

[11] Reyes Guillén I, Sánchez-Pérez HJ, Cruz-Burguete JL, de Izaurieta M. Anti-tuberculosis treatment defaulting. An analysis of perceptions and interactions in Chiapas, Mexico. Salud Publica Mex 2008; 58(3)251-257.

[12] Sánchez-Pérez HJ, Díaz-Vázquez A, Nájera-Ortíz JC, Balandrano S, Martín-Mateo M. Multidrug-resistant pulmonary tuberculosis in Los Altos, Selva and Norte regions of Chiapas, Mexico. Int J Tuber Lung Dis 2010;14(1):34-39.

[13] Nájera-Ortiz JC, Sánchez-Pérez HJ, Ochoa-Díaz H, Arana-Cedeño M, Salazar Lezama MA, Martín Mateo M. Demographic, health services and socio-economic factors associated with pulmonary tuberculosis mortality in Los Altos Region of Chiapas, Mexico. International Journal of Epidemiology 2008;37:786-795.

[14] Najera-Ortiz JC, Sánchez-Pérez HJ, Ochoa-Díaz-López H, Leal-Fernández G, and Navarro i Gine A. The poor survival among pulmonary tuberculosis patients in Chiapas, Mexico: The Case of Los Altos Region. Tuberculosis Research and Treatment. doi:10.1155/2012/708423 (accessed 12 August 2012).

[15] Sistema Integrado de Indicadores Sociales del Ecuador (SIISE) EcoCIENCIA, 2005. Socio-Environmental Monitoring System of Cotopaxi Province, Ecuador: SIISE; 2007.

[16] Romero Sandoval N, Flores Carrera O, Sánchez Pérez HJ, Sánchez Pérez I, Martín Mateo M. Pulmonary tuberculosis in an indigenous community of the mountains of Ecuador. Int J Tuber Lung Dis 2007;11(5)550-555.

[17] Romero-Sandoval N, Flores-Carrera O, Molina MA, Jácome M, Navarro A, Martín. DOTS strategy and community participation: an experience in the Ecuatorian Andes. Int J Tuberc Lung Dis 2009;13(12):1569-1571.

[18] Horna-Campos O, Sánchez-Pérez HJ, Sánchez-Pérez I, Bedoya Lama A, Martín Mateo M. Public transportation and pulmonary tuberculosis, Lima, Peru. Emerging Infectious Diseases 2007;13(10):1491-1493.

[19] Horna-Campos OJ, Consiglio E, Sánchez-Pérez HJ, Navarro A, Caylá JA, Martín-Mateo M. Pulmonary tuberculosis infection among workers in the informal public transport sector in Lima Peru. Occup Environ Med 2011; 68:163-165.

[20] Horna-Campos, O.J, Bedoya-Lama, A, Romero-Sandoval, N, Martín-Mateo, M. Risk of tuberculosis in public transport sector workers, Lima, Peru. Int J Tuberc Lung Dis 2010; 14 (6): 714-719.

[21] United Nations, Department of Public Information. The United Nations today. New York: United Nations 2008.

[22] Lönnroth K, Jaramillo E, Williams BG, Dye C, Raviglione M. Drivers of tuberculosis epidemics: The role of risk factors and social determinants. Social Science & Medicine 2009; 68: 2240–2246.

[23] Donald P, Van Helden P. The Global Burden of Tuberculosis — Combating Drug. Resistance in Difficult Times. N Engl J Med 2009; 360(23): 2393-2395.

[24] Benatar S. R., Upshur R. Tuberculosis and poverty: what could (and should) be done? Int J Tuberc Lung Dis 2010; 14(10):1215–1221. http://www.ifaisa.org/current_affairs/The_year_of_the_lung.pdf (accessed 11 August 2012).

[25] Montero E, Zapata EM, Vázquez V, Nazar A, Sánchez-Pérez HJ. Tuberculosis en la Sierra Santa Marta, Veracruz: un análisis desde la perspectiva de género. Papeles de población 2001; 29: 225-245.

[26] Andrulis DP. Access to care is the centrepiece in the elimination of socioeconomic disparities in health. Ann Intern Med 1998;129:412-416.

[27] Saver B, Peterfreund N. Insurance, income and access to health care. JAMA 1995;275:305-11.

[28] Zignol M, Gemert W, Falzon D, Sismanidis Ch, Glaziou Ph, Floyd K, Raviglione M. Surveillance of anti-tuberculosis drug resistance in the world: an updated analysis 2007-2010. Bull World Health Organ 2012; 90(2):111-119D. doi: 10.2471/BLT.11.092585 (accessed 11 August 2012).

[29] Instituto Nacional de Estadística, Geografía e Informática (INEGI). Statistical Year-book Chiapas 2004. Aguascalientes: INEGI, México; 2004.

[30] Ticona E. Tuberculosis: Se agotó el enfoque biomédico. Revista Peruana de Medicina Experimental y Salud Pública 2009; 26:273-275.

[31] Arana-Cedeño M. Dos padecimientos de la pobreza y la exclusión en Chiapas: la des-nutrición y la tuberculosis. In: Pérez Arguelles M (Coord). Cinco miradas sobre el derecho a la salud. Estudios de caso en México, El Salvador y Nicaragua. México, D.F.: Fundar, Centro de Análisis e Investigación, A.C; 2010. p177-230.

[32] Estrella E. Diagnóstico y tratamiento. In: Estrella E. La medicina en el Ecuador pre-hispánico. Quito, Ecuador: Casa de la Cultura Ecuatoriana 'Benjamín Carrión', Fondo Editorial CCE; 2006. p209-230.

[33] Page J. El mandato de los dioses. Etnomedicina entre los tzotziles de Chamula y Che-nalhó, Chiapas. México, D.F.: Programa de Investigaciones Multidisciplinarias sobre Mesoamérica y El Sureste, Instituto de Investigaciones Antropológicas, Universidad Nacional Autónoma de México (PROIMMSE-IIA-UNAM), Colección científica 11; 2005.

[34] Mendoza A, Gotuzo E. Tuberculosis extremadamente resistente (TB-XDR): historia y situación actual. Acta Médica Peruana 2008; 25:236-246.

[35] Sánchez-Pérez HJ, Halperin D. Problemas de diagnóstico de la tuberculosis pulmo-nar. El caso de la región fronteriza de Chiapas. Atención Primaria 1997; 19(5): 237-242.

[36] Ryan F. The forgotten plague – how the battle against tuberculosis was won and lost. Boston, Mass: Lost Back Books; 1993.

[37] World Health Organization (WHO). How health systems can address inequities in priority public health conditions: the example of tuberculosis. Geneva: WHO; 2010.

[38] Alvarez-Gordillo G, Dorantes-Jiménez J, Molina-Rosales D. La búsqueda de atención para la tuberculosis en Chiapas, México. Rev Panam salud Publica/Pan Am J Public Health 2001; 9(5): 285-293.

[39] Galtung J. Violence, peace, and peace research. Journal of Peace Research 1969; 6:167-191.

[40] McKeown T, Record RG. Reason for the decline of mortality in England and Wales during the nineteenth century. Population Studies 1962; 16: 94-122.

[41] Commission on Social Determinants for Health. Closing the gap in a generation: Health equity through action on the social determinants of health. Final report of the Commission on Social Determinants of Health. Geneva: World Health Organization; 2008.

[42] World Health Organization (WHO). Instrumentos Internacionales de Derechos Humanos. HRI/GEN/Rev.5, 26 de abril. Recopilación de las Observaciones Generales y Recomendaciones generales Adoptadas por Órganos Creados en virtud de Tratados de Derechos Humanos. http://servindi.org/pdf/ObservacionesyRecomendacionesGenerales.pdf (accessed 8 July 2012).

[43] United Nations Committee Economic, Social and Cultural Rights (UN CESCR). General Comment 14. Geneva: UN CESCR; 2000.

[44] Veneklasen L, Miller V, Clark C, and Reilly M. Rights-based approaches and beyond: Challenges of linking rights and participation. Brighton, Sussex: Institute of Development Studies (IDS). Working Paper 235, December 2004:13-17.

[45] International Labour Organization. Convention No. 169, Art. 25.

[46] UN CESCR. General Comment 4: The Nature of States Parties Obligations. UN doc E/1991/23. Geneva: 14 December 1990, Annex III, paragraph 10.

Permissions

The contributors of this book come from diverse backgrounds, making this book a truly international effort. This book will bring forth new frontiers with its revolutionizing research information and detailed analysis of the nascent developments around the world.

We would like to thank Dr. Bassam H. Mahboub and Dr. Mayank G. Vats, for lending their expertise to make the book truly unique. They have played a crucial role in the development of this book. Without their invaluable contribution this book wouldn't have been possible. They have made vital efforts to compile up to date information on the varied aspects of this subject to make this book a valuable addition to the collection of many professionals and students.

This book was conceptualized with the vision of imparting up-to-date information and advanced data in this field. To ensure the same, a matchless editorial board was set up. Every individual on the board went through rigorous rounds of assessment to prove their worth. After which they invested a large part of their time researching and compiling the most relevant data for our readers. Conferences and sessions were held from time to time between the editorial board and the contributing authors to present the data in the most comprehensible form. The editorial team has worked tirelessly to provide valuable and valid information to help people across the globe.

Every chapter published in this book has been scrutinized by our experts. Their significance has been extensively debated. The topics covered herein carry significant findings which will fuel the growth of the discipline. They may even be implemented as practical applications or may be referred to as a beginning point for another development. Chapters in this book were first published by InTech; hereby published with permission under the Creative Commons Attribution License or equivalent.

The editorial board has been involved in producing this book since its inception. They have spent rigorous hours researching and exploring the diverse topics which have resulted in the successful publishing of this book. They have passed on their knowledge of decades through this book. To expedite this challenging task, the publisher supported the team at every step. A small team of assistant editors was also appointed to further simplify the editing procedure and attain best results for the readers.

Our editorial team has been hand-picked from every corner of the world. Their multi-ethnicity adds dynamic inputs to the discussions which result in innovative outcomes. These outcomes are then further discussed with the researchers and contributors who give their valuable feedback and opinion regarding the same. The feedback is then collaborated with the researches and they are edited in a comprehensive manner to aid the understanding of the subject.

Apart from the editorial board, the designing team has also invested a significant amount of their time in understanding the subject and creating the most relevant covers. They scrutinized every image to scout for the most suitable representation of the subject and create an appropriate cover for the book.

The publishing team has been involved in this book since its early stages. They were actively engaged in every process, be it collecting the data, connecting with the contributors or procuring relevant information. The team has been an ardent support to the editorial, designing and production team. Their endless efforts to recruit the best for this project, has resulted in the accomplishment of this book. They are a veteran in the field of academics and their pool of knowledge is as vast as their experience in printing. Their expertise and guidance has proved useful at every step. Their uncompromising quality standards have made this book an exceptional effort. Their encouragement from time to time has been an inspiration for everyone.

The publisher and the editorial board hope that this book will prove to be a valuable piece of knowledge for researchers, students, practitioners and scholars across the globe.

List of Contributors

Simona Alexandra Iacob
National Institute of Infectious Diseases "Matei Bals" Bucharest, Romania

Diana Gabriela Iacob
"Carol Davila" University of Medicine and Pharmacie, Bucharest, Romania

Wolfgang Frank
Lungenklinik Amsee, Waren (Müritz), Germany

Claude Kirimuhuzya
Department of Pharmacology and Toxicology, Faculty of Biomedical Sciences, Kampala International University-Western Campus, Bushenyi, Uganda

Juan D. Guzman
Subdirección de Investigación, Instituto Nacional de Salud, Bogotá, Colombia

Ximena Montes-Rincón and Wellman Ribón
Grupo de Inmunología y Epidemiologia Molecular, Universidad Industrial de Santander, Bucaramanga, Colombia

Marcos Catanho
Laboratory for Functional Genomics and Bioinformatics, Oswaldo Cruz Institute, Rio de Janeiro, Brazil

Antonio Basílio de Miranda
Laboratory of Computational Biology and Systems, Oswaldo Cruz Institute, Rio de Janeiro, Brazil

Luciene C. Scherer
Lutheran University of Brasil-ULBRA, Canoas/ RS/, Brazil

Héctor Javier Sánchez-Pérez
Society, Culture and Health Academic Area, The College of the Southern Border (ECOSUR), San Cristóbal de Las Casas, Chiapas, The Africa and Latin America Research Groups Network (GRAAL)-ECOSUR, Mexico

Olivia Horna–Campos
The Africa and Latin America Research Groups Network (GRAAL), Faculty of Medicine, Biostatistics Unit, Barcelona Autonomous University, Bellaterra, Spain
Barcelona Public Health Agency, Epidemiology Service, Barcelona, Spain

Natalia Romero-Sandoval
School of Medicine, Pontificia Universidad Católica del Ecuador, Quito, The Africa and Latin America Research Groups Network - GRAAL-ECUADOR, Ecuador

Ezequiel Consiglio
Society, Culture and Health Academic Area, The College of the Southern Border (ECOSUR), San Cristóbal de Las Casas, Chiapas, The Africa and Latin America Research Groups Network (GRAAL)-ECOSUR, Mexico
University Institute of Health, National University of La Matanza, San Justo, Buenos Aires, Argentina

Miguel Martín Mateo
The Africa and Latin America Research Groups Network (GRAAL). Faculty of Medicine, Biostatistics Unit, Barcelona Autonomous University, Bellaterra, Spain